The Raw Secrets

The Raw Food Diet in the Real World

By Frédéric Patenaude
www.fredericpatenaude.com

Disclaimer

The responsibility for any consequences resulting from any suggestion or procedure described hereafter does not lie with the author, publisher or distributors of this book. This book is not intended as medical advice.

Copyright Information

Cover art: Martin Mailloux

First Edition, October 2002

ISBN-10:   1-449-55845-3
ISBN-13:   978-1-449558-45-1

Second edition: April 2006

If you would like to publish sections of this book, please contact the publisher.

Published by:

FredericPatenaude.Com
6595 St-Hubert, CP 59053
Montreal (Quebec)
H2S 3P5, Canada
www.fredericpatenaude.com

To register your copy of this book and access your free book bonuses, go to:
www.rawsecretsbonus.com

Some Letters Received
Since publication of 1st Edition
of *The Raw Secrets*

"I got *The Raw Secrets* yesterday and spent all day today reading it. It was absolutely genius, yet simple!

I started eating 100% raw in January. It solved years of problems, but only lasted three months. Then, many of the problems mentioned in your book crept in... without my really being aware of them. I knew the diet was right, but something was wrong...such frustrating and unnerving feelings!

I prayed that God would open my eyes and lead me to the right sources of information on this topic (since there is so much contradictory information out there.) That very day I ran across your website. After reading many of the articles, I decided to order your book *The Raw Secrets*. It was very impressive and inspiring and an answer to my prayer!

I know I have a lot more research and experimentation to do, but your book greatly helped to steer me in a positive and promising direction!

Thank you so much for all the time you put into this book! God bless your efforts as you continue to research, experiment and share what you know! This information is incredible... just truly awesome!"

Erica Ormonde
Baker City, OR USA

"I just finished *The Raw Secrets* and I want to thank you for writing it. You have done the burgeoning raw food movement a great service by pointing out the mistakes of raw-fooders and exposing misconceptions that would lead them to failure."

Nora Lenz
Bellevue, Washington

"Hi, I got the book *The Raw Secrets* and thoroughly enjoyed it. I've already read it twice and I wish I had read it a long time ago. I've been trying to go raw for a year and have had all the problems you described in your book. Thanks so much for writing the book!"

Leatha Day

"Your latest book *The Raw Secrets* became available just in time to clear the path ahead for me. I was truly drowning in misinformation."

Tom Szelagowski

"I've just finished The Raw Secrets — the best 'raw' book I've read so far. Great work! Can't wait for your next book!

Joanne Scovill
Middletown

"It is the best and most down-to-earth book on the raw lifestyle that I've ever read. My girlfriend and I read it more than once. I will most certainly recommend it to anyone."

Brian Dallas
Texas

"The confusion in the raw food community is vast. I thank you for your clarity and research."

Bill Seaberry
Mt. Shasta, California

"I wanted to tell you how much I enjoyed your book. I think that you included a lot of very useful information that I probably would have never known about."

Shari Vermeulen

"Your book *The Raw Secrets* has been very helpful to me and I wanted to tell you how much I appreciate all your work. At first, I was skeptical because you are so young (I am 55) and then I realized that you had no doubt done a lot more in the "raw food eating" department than I, so your age certainly did not matter. I love the raw food way of eating for its simplicity and ease, but your book gave me the added confidence and explained many of the mistakes that I can now avoid. The planet needs more people like you!"

L. Rebecca Perry
Houston, Texas

"I am reading your new book *The Raw Secrets* and am really enjoying the groundedness you are bringing to the raw food movement through this book."

Mark O'Connor
Berkeley, CA

"I've just finished your book, *The Raw Secrets* and would like to say it's a fantastically great book. I have been a fruitarian/raw foodist for about 10 years now, and have made so many mistakes along the way, some up until just today. There are many "Eurekas" in your book that explain so much."

Sidnumber

"I just finished reading your new book a few days ago, and I absolutely love it! It was definitely very motivating. I have been doing the raw food diet for about 3 months now and have made some of the mistakes you have talked about in the book."

Angela Brasier

"I received the book *The Raw Secrets*. It makes a lot of sense and it seems like it is speaking directly to me. I really appreciate the insights. I am very optimistic with what this book has taught me thus far."

Brian

"I am just in the midst of reading your book *The Raw Secrets*. I must say that I am thrilled that someone else out there has had the same experience I have been having and had the courage to go public with it!

Karen

"I began reading *The Raw Secrets* and was impressed with the fact that you share your vulnerabilities and past difficulties with raw food eating. This alone provides invaluable information for your readers.

I've been researching the raw food idea for quite some time and recently determined that Raw Secrets was the book I needed to cut through the crap and get to the heart of what I needed to know. As you wrote, 'This is the book I wish someone had handed to me six years ago...' I want to express my gratitude to you for having written *Raw Secrets* so I won't have to wish. ;-)

Marcus
Montreal, Canada

"My name is Misgana Isaak, and I just bought your book and fell in love with it. I feel like you just wrote this book for me."

Misgana Isaak

"I am really glad I bought your book *The Raw Secrets*. There is so much practical advice and reading in words what I was already instinctively feeling has been very important. It is so non-mainstream that it is sometimes difficult to trust my own inner intuition!! Many thanks. I'm already reading some parts for the third time. I seem to find new gems each time."

Jayne Jubb

"I received your book yesterday from Amazon.com and read it. Awesome. In the past year or so I've just been reading a lot of books and getting the logistics of food purchase and prep planning. I am sure glad for your book. Thanks for being practical, truthful, and honest and telling it like it is. Now I know I can do this. You rock. Keep up the good work."

John Schmidt
Portland

Acknowledgments, 1ˢᵗ Edition, *The Raw Secrets*

Special thanks to **Albert Mosséri** for letting me translate his writings. Without his knowledge, this work would not have been possible.

Special thanks to **Andrew Durham**, who edited the first edition of *The Raw Secrets*. Many thanks for your insights, which helped clarify many areas in this book, and also for your constant support to this project.

I would like to thank all the people who have directly or indirectly contributed to the realization of this book:

Marianne Moineau for her constant support and belief in this project, our long conversations and experiments that have helped me formulate my thoughts and ideas, and her help in the realization of this project.

Olivier Magnan for the initial motivation and idea that led to the creation of this book. C'était ton idée!

Fabi Reaume for much-needed proofreading.

Beata Barinbaum for last-minute critique of the book and proofreading.

Robert Harrison for help in proofreading the book.

The Boutenko Family for some last minute, raw inspiration! Spasibo!

David Norman for support through the years of all of my endeavors.

Enrique Candioti for the raw inspiration and help with the magazine.

Paul Nison, whose approach to the raw food diet has helped me formulate many areas of this book.
Dr. Doug Graham, whose research has helped me clarify my thinking in many areas of this book.
Dr. Fred Bisci, whose insights have helped me formulate some areas of this book.
Louiselle Houle, pour avoir procuré un endroit où rester durant les débuts de ce projet.
Réal Patenaude, qui m'a toujours encouragé dans mes projets.
Sébastien Patenaude for being part of my first raw experiences and the support (ça aide d'avoir un frère.)

Acknowledgments, 2nd Edition, *The Raw Secrets*

Rob Miller for help in editing the 2nd edition.
Ela for your help in editing the second edition of this book. Many thanks!
Kathy Raine for your help in editing the final touches of this second edition.

TABLE OF CONTENTS

INTRODUCTION
In the Raw

Radical ideas have much more power than common advice. But in their power lies the danger. Like an explosive charge, radical ideas must be handled carefully.

The raw vegan diet is such an idea. It can save your life. It can help banish "incurable" conditions. It can help you feel great all the time. It can give back your joy of living. It can give an entirely different direction to your life or turn it upside down.

But the practical application may be difficult. Pitfalls line the path of raw eating. Many people have fallen into them — and they will continue falling into them until they know what these pitfalls are, and how to spot and avoid them.

Some people are damaging their health by eating the raw food diet incorrectly. Mostly, this is because they received poor or confusing advice. This book is my antidote to the false information that is being spread in the raw food movement, hurting people as it goes. This is the book I wish someone had handed to me in 1997 when I started on this path.

My dietary adventures have led me to write *The Raw Secrets*. Even though I had experienced benefits in eating a raw food diet immediately, my personal experience with it has not been an instant success story. It has been one of the most positive things I have ever undertaken — but it has also been a struggle. So before revealing my findings, I wish to share with you my story.

I became aware of the link between diet and health at the age of 16, when my mother introduced vegetarianism into my family. She had decided to make some changes in her diet in order to lose some weight. Suddenly, whole wheat bread, tofu, seitan and other strange items made their appearance in our fridge. Meat slowly disappeared.

My mom's interest in nutrition quickly spread to me as I started to read the books on the subject that she had bought. I gradually became a vegetarian without calling myself one. A couple years later, the final blow came when I read the book *Diet For a New America,* by John Robbins. It convinced me to become a vegetarian and gave me all the right reasons to do so.

Vegetarianism was fun for me. I remember the excitement of discovering all these new products; of shopping at health food stores for the first time; of learning to make new foods; and of trying to impose my new beliefs on friends and family at the first opportunity. It was fun. But vegetarianism didn't turn my world upside down.

Raw food did.

By chance I found a little book by Herbert Shelton called *Food Combining Made Easy.* It made a strong impression on me. Shelton stated that humans, like other frugivorous animals on the planet, are meant to live on fruits, vegetables, nuts, seeds and nothing else. For a grain-based vegetarian, this statement drilled a big hole into my comfortable, newly found vegetarian box. I thought I had found the ultimate diet. But here comes this guy saying that not only would I have to give up meat and dairy, but also grains, beans, oils, salt, seasonings, as well as everything cooked and processed! I felt assaulted. I thought that I had to find out more about this stuff, because it couldn't possibly be right.

On the same shelf where I found Shelton's works, I came across some strange-looking books in French by a gentleman named Albert Mosséri. I was shocked to discover that he was saying the same thing. Our natural diet should be composed of fruits and vegetables, and maybe some nuts and seeds.

Beyond these matters of content and instruction, these books on *Natural Hygiene* were saying that each of us is solely responsible for his or her health. They stated that all the sickness we experience is the result of wrong living -- primarily the wrong diet. And that by returning to a simple raw food diet of fruits and vegetables, with fasting (if necessary), we could not only heal from all these diseases, but we could also go back to our pristine, natural state -- nothing less than exuberant health.

So, I kept reading more about *Natural Hygiene*. I remember the feelings I had looking at the photo on the cover of Mosséri's book. In the photo there was a bowl of fruit, a few chestnuts, and a strange looking squash. It seemed so austere, yet so attractive. I remember the conflict that went on inside of me. I know this is for real. What these people are saying makes a lot of sense. But then to actually do this requires that I change my life around and take it in a completely different direction than what I had planned." That's what a twenty-year-old guy was going through somewhere in Quebec, Canada. And I thought I was all-alone.

So I went into this on my own, and without much success. I kept going back and forth. My diet was chaotic, and too much had been stirred up inside of me that I didn't know how to handle it. I needed to meet some new people, to get the hell out of my hometown, and find out what was going on elsewhere. So one night on the Internet I found out about a book called *Nature's First Law: The Raw Food Diet* by Arlin, Dini, and Wolfe.

Nature's First Law seriously motivated me to go all-raw. I got in contact with the authors in San Diego and arranged for a meeting. I went all-raw for six months in Canada, got a couple of friends into it, and worked to save money at the same time. Then I packed my stuff, since I needed to take my time to absorb all of this, and boarded a 72-hour, six-layover bus to California.

In California, I found the raw-food movement fresh and young, but also confusing and full of contradictions. I found myself going along with the wave, being part of what was happening. Along the way I got the idea that the raw food diet was the answer to everything. I thought that it would not only solve all of my problems, but it would, in the long run, also solve all of humanity's problems. Perhaps this enthusiasm was necessary to get me started (like many others, I'm sure), but it certainly was misleading.

In California, although I was trying to maintain an air of balance and enthusiasm, my health was going slowly downhill. Too bad for a young guy like me! I found that I was constantly running out of energy. Often I felt spacey, unable to concentrate and unable to find the energy needed to go on with normal daily activities. I thought I was going through a detox and that this would stop one day — that I would finally feel "paradise health". Unfortunately, that day never came. The "detox" was never-ending.

Behind the scenes, seeds and fats were taking over my diet. I was sometimes eating five to six avocados a day, as well as a lot of nuts and seeds. To pacify my cravings, I began to use oil, condiments, salt, garlic and other items that I had previously eschewed following *Natural Hygiene* in Canada. Since the last thing I wanted to do was eat cooked food, I created all sorts of replacements for the cooked foods I was craving. I went berserk with raw food recipes: raw pies, raw chocolate, raw lasagna, you name it. All raw. All organic. All healthy…right? But…

After a year, I got really sick for an entire month. But I told nobody, because I was this great raw-foodist and I was supposed to be incredibly healthy. I wasn't supposed to get sick like that. So I hid at home and fasted until I felt better.

After that experience, things became clearer. I realized that the raw diet regime couldn't be followed haphazardly. I was still clueless about how to do it. Excluding nuts from my diet for a while after the fast really helped, but I was still far from "paradise health". Where was the boundless energy to dance all night? Where had the fire gone?

To top it off, I was this guy working at Nature's First Law, *world headquarters of the raw food diet*. There, I had started my own raw newsletter, *Just Eat An Apple*, and I was on my way to writing a recipe book, having become quite a good raw chef along the way.

During these first few years I wasn't always drained, but for a big chunk of my time as a strict raw-foodist in California I was trying to figure out why this wasn't really working for me the way it was supposed to, according to the books. And I was not alone. I was meeting a lot of other people going through the same thing. But clouded by the ideal of raw-foodism, we wouldn't admit to ourselves what was happening.

When I moved back to Canada in 2000, I'd had it. I started eating cooked food again, and – incredibly enough – I started feeling better. I started feeling better because I had stepped back from my position of being a strict raw-foodist and was able to see the raw food diet for what it was. I saw it as a tool, one that could be used poorly, or one that could be used properly. I just hadn't learned how to use it properly yet.

Because I am given to excess, I re-explored the cooked diet just as fully as I had explored the raw food diet. Slowly and carefully, I tested cooked food on my body. I tried bread. I tried cheese. On dates at restaurants, I drank wine. I felt what it is like to order a croissant in a café in Paris. I realized that I had changed my body so much by eating a raw food diet that I could no longer eat the stuff I used to and feel "normal" like "normal people". My body reacted strongly and rejected these foods. I needed to find something, and fast, because I knew that eating like this wasn't for me.

Back to square one, I rediscovered *Natural Hygiene*. I carefully reread Mosséri's and Shelton's books, the ones I read before I went to California. These books had turned my life upside down and gave me the courage to go live somewhere else for two and a half years with only $600 in my bank account.

Having gathered all that experience, this time I could fully grasp the basic principles of health delineated by Mosséri. I could see them at work in everything that had happened to others and to me. I was able to see what had gone wrong for me and why. Through this new understanding, I was able to really experience the benefits that were promised to me by the early leaders of the raw-food movement.

To get back to the raw food diet, I began with small steps. First, I found that the most important thing was to eat mostly foods that are biologically specific to human beings: fruits, vegetables, and *small* quantities of nuts and seeds; and avoiding grains, beans and condiments. I had to pay attention to hunger, food combinations, and the quantities of fat, nuts and seeds in my diet. I also found that when eating baked roots or steamed vegetables, I felt much better than when I was eating lots of nuts and seeds or complicated raw recipes.

This book is a summation of the secrets I have discovered about the raw food diet. Each chapter contains a lesson, a message to *myself* about the subject that helped me see the whole picture again. Some of the chapters are combative, reflecting the struggles I went through. Some are more positive, reflecting the insights that occurred to me.

I understood that the raw food diet is not so simple to put into practice. You can very easily damage your health eating a raw food diet, probably without being aware of it at first. If you're new to it, you can count yourself lucky to have found this book. There's a lot of misleading advice out there, and I'm glad you've found the right guide first.

My main problem for many years was a lack of energy. I often felt drained, even though I was eating the best foods in the world. It took me a long time to figure out what was going on. Unfortunately, the only advice I received from raw-foodists was, "Keep on eating raw until you get through the Detox."

I have met all sorts of people doing this diet, from the sensible to the fanatical and everything in between. I met some people who ate what they called a Raw Food Diet for many years and then went back to bread and meat. Others who had sworn in the name of Raw that they'd never go back to cooked food were later found enjoying hot bean burritos without a sign of guilt. How did this happen?

Some people tend to quickly figure it out on their own. For them, it takes four days to see what others like me take four years to sort out. Their reason and intuition are in good order. But imbalanced or extreme people (a lot of us) don't find it so easy, especially when our only guides are a few books filled with wrong advice. Sadly, most of the books on the raw food diet fit this description. I offer *The Raw Secrets* as a good guide to the raw food diet.

Just as the book *Fit For Life* misled people years ago, making them believe that they were practicing *Natural Hygiene* just because they were combining bread or chicken properly, new raw-foodists on the scene are being misled into thinking that they are eating a healthy raw food diet just because the foods they eat are unheated.

There are plenty of ideas and talk but a lack of facts and wisdom. There is definitely a lack of basic principles. And this leads to major confusion. When people go to raw-food festivals or raw-food conferences, they come home very inspired, and sometimes also very confused. Why? Because although all the speakers promote a raw food diet, they disagree on what it consists of. One says that fruit is the best of all foods, another says that fruit feeds internal mold. One promotes supplements, while another says that no supplements should ever be consumed. One guy recommends water fasting, while the other says it is dangerous and that we should take juices instead. And so on. All this confusion exists because most raw-foodists — teachers and students alike — are unaware of the basic principles of health. The lack of basic principles in any science will lead to its disintegration. This lack is particularly obvious in the raw food movement, whose leaders cannot agree among them on what constitutes the raw food diet.

Nonetheless, these basic principles do exist. They were rediscovered 170 years ago by the *Natural Hygienist*s in the United States, and by the members of the German back-to-nature movement. In this book, I present some of the basic principles of *Natural Hygiene* and how they apply to the raw food diet, undermining some raw mythology along the way.

This is pretty new stuff for most of us, and we're bound to make mistakes and commit excesses, even *heinous* ones. But at the end of the mistakes comes a period of ordering and cleaning up, and the first part of cleaning is taking out the garbage.

For many people, raw-foodism has become a sort of religion where cooked food is evil and raw food is salvation. Many books have exaggerated the benefits offered by the raw food diet and neglected its practical application. Some raw-foodists even think that anything raw is better than anything cooked. They think that all they need to do is to eat raw foods and avoid cooked foods at all costs. However, as many have discovered the hard way, health and natural diet are not so simple.

An old saying goes, "Better is often the enemy of the good." In common parlance, we say that someone "can't see the forest for the trees." By trying to be too perfect, you can sometimes lose your mind. Many raw-foodists, including myself, have promoted the concept that my friend, Dr. Doug Graham, calls the *Raw/Not Raw Philosophy*. It is an oversimplification of all health principles into one criterion: "Is this raw?" Rather than wondering, "Is this healthy for me?" or "What do I experience in my body after eating this?" Some raw-foodists only want to know, "Is this raw?" For vegans, the question is, "Is it vegan?"

An adherent of the *Raw/Not Raw Philosophy* would, for example, shun steamed vegetables, but will not hesitate to eat a jar of raw almond butter in a week, or even in a day. He eschews all cooked food, never thinking that some of his 'raw' eating habits could harm him more than some 'cooked' diet plans. A convinced vegan will avoid all animal products, but he or she might use salt, oils, sugar and processed foods out of a factory, as long as they are "vegan".

Natural nutrition asks for more clarity. Raw-foodism is not a religion. How you eat should be based on rational principles of physiology, not an over-simplified mantra.

Raw-foodism and veganism are valid, but not the way they are sometimes practiced, especially these days. In this book, you will learn how to eat a raw food diet in a way that is sustainable and vitalizing.

Frédéric Patenaude
October, 2002, revised March 2006
Montreal, Quebec, Canada

CHAPTER 1

How to Determine Our Natural Diet

The first question we need to answer before going any further, before talking about raw food or cooked food, is the following: What foods are biologically specific to the human body?

This question can also be phrased in another way: What is our natural diet as humans?

The Biological Approach

Nutritionists would like to determine our diet according to various tests, chemical analysis and research done in laboratories, and define the exact proportions of nutrients we need. They would then come up with a formula with how much zinc a person needs every day, how much calcium, and so on. Eventually a person following this biochemical approach to nutrition ends up eating according to charts. They eat this food for calcium, that food for iron, they make sure they take in this quantity of that supplement, while ingesting other pills and powders to make sure they get everything they "need". That leads to the idea of the "balanced diet", *which no animal in nature follows.*

On top of that, the various researchers don't agree with each other on the exact quantities of nutrients needed and where to get them. Eventually, nutrition gets so complicated that it makes everybody wonder, "How do we know what to eat?" It seems as if eating, which is the most natural thing to do, is something so complicated that only an expert with a degree can tell us how to do it, based on research done in laboratories.

Whenever someone tells me "Nutrition is so complicated," I respond, "It doesn't seem to be for the animals in the wild." I remind them that wild animals do not think of nutrition as anything complex. They simplify the matter by eating only raw, natural foods for which they are biologically designed.

Laboratory tests and analysis will never be able to determine accurately what we should eat, because this approach to nutrition is a complete departure from the natural way. What natural hygienists of the past have done instead is use the *biological approach*. In this approach, we try to define the place of humans in nature in the dietetic field. We try to determine if we're carnivores, herbivores, omnivores or simply frugivores. Once we've established our dietetic nature, it becomes easy to determine what foods constitute the best sources of human nourishment.

The rational approach to nutrition, the one I have followed in this book, is as follows:

1) *First, determine our natural diet*: What foods are we biologically designed to eat?
2) *Second, pay attention to all of the factors that can get in the way of optimal nutrition.* Secure enough sleep, engage in physical activity, avoid unhealthy habits (coffee, drugs, alcohol, medicines, etc.)
3) *Third, eat foods as close to nature as possible.* This means eating raw, unprocessed, unseasoned, whole foods.

The Logical Approach

The author and researcher Herbert Shelton describes how one of his predecessors, Dr. Densmore, tried to define our natural diet:

> In his efforts to establish, to his

complete satisfaction, the normal diet of
man, Dr. Emmet Densmore pursued a line
of reasoning that we may consider with
profit. First he noted that animals in
their natural state live upon foods that
are spontaneously produced by nature, and
require no cultivation. Man, on the other
hand, he noted, lives upon foods that are
produced by cultivation. Man does not live
upon the spontaneous products of nature,
but lives artificially.

The thought then occurred to him that, if
nature has provided a *natural food* for all
the animals below man, perhaps she has also
provided a normal food for man. He assumed
that nature has produced foods that are
as normal to man as grasses are to the
herbivore, or as flesh is to the carnivore.
This was certainly no unreasonable
assumption, but is based on the principles
of the unity of nature. It is based upon
the fact that man, as much as the lion or
the deer, is a child of nature and that,
like these animals, his normal requirements
are found in nature. If man, like the other
animals of nature, is constituted for a
certain type of food, what is that food or
what is that type? What, in other words,
is the normal food of man? He sought his
answers in several directions. Scientists
agreed that man's original home was in a
warm climate, either in the tropics or the
sub-tropics. Without tools and without fire,
he must have lived in a part of the world
where the spontaneous productions of nature
could be obtained by him with only the
"tools" with which he is physiologically
equipped and could eat without artificial
preparation.

```
If man first lived in a warm climate," he
reasoned, "and if like other animals, he
subsisted on foods spontaneously produced
by nature, these foods must have been
those which grow wild in such a climate,
quite probably such foods as are still
spontaneously produced in such localities.
The woods of the south, as is well-known,
abound in sweet fruits and nuts."

It will be seen at a glance that this line
of reasoning led straight to the fruits of
the trees as man's normal diet.
          Herbert Shelton, in Hygienic
          Review, July 1971
```

Let's add to this fascinating exposé by Shelton the fact that nuts are only available for part of the year in warm climates. And they are available fresh, not dried. Also, vegetables and vegetable matter abound all year round and have probably been consumed by humans for as long as they have been on this planet.

Let's also consider the fact that, since the beginning of agriculture, humans have been cultivating -- and eating -- foodstuffs that they are not necessarily designed to eat, notably grains. This also means that we have stopped propagating the wild fruits that once made up the largest part of our diet (i.e. because we've been eating less of them.) Because of this, if you were to go wander in most tropical jungles of the world, you would be surprised to find how little food there is to eat!

There are some places, though, where a huge variety of the most amazing fruits still grow in the wild. These places are the jungles in South-East Asia, where some of the great apes live. When animals like a fruit, or any other natural food, they eat it and carry the swallowed seeds inside them to excrete elsewhere, thus propagating the species of the fruit they prefer. Thus they create, after hundreds of years, the food environment best suited to them. Since our tastes are still very close to theirs, it's only in the regions where the primates live that we may find an abundance of edible, wild fruits.

What is our place in nature?

> Every anatomical, physiological and embryological feature of man definitely places him in the class Frugivore. The number and structure of his teeth, the length and structure of his digestive tract, the position of his eyes, the character of his nails, the functions of his skin, the character of his saliva, the relative size of his liver, the number and position of the milk glands, the position and structure of the sexual organs, the character of the human placenta and many other factors all bear witness to the fact that man is constitutionally a frugivore.
>
> As there are no pure frugivores, all frugivores eating freely of green leaves and other parts of plants, man may, also, without violating his constitutional nature, partake of green plants. These parts of plants possess certain advantages, as has been previously pointed out, in which fruits are deficient. Actual tests have shown that the addition of green vegetables to the fruit and nut diet improves the diet.
> *Shelton, Orthotrophy.*

Nature is not in chaos. When we look at the different animals in nature, we can see that each of them has been designed to eat a particular diet — to thrive on particular foods. The diet of animals is usually restricted to a few categories of foods only. And those foods are the ones they have been designed to process the best.

Let's just take a look at our teeth. It is widely accepted by biologists that the form and shape of teeth is of great importance when classifying animals. Even the primates, whose diet consists chiefly of fruits and vegetables with a very small amount of animal products, have teeth that are more appropriate than ours to eating meat.

But open the mouth of your cat or dog and notice the long canines. They are conical and sharp. Those canines can lock into each other, on each side of the mouth. Now take a look at your own canines. They're barely sharp enough to bite into an apple! Even if you try to bite your own finger with those canines, I guarantee that you won't be able to cut yourself and make yourself bleed. Now don't let your dog try the same on you!

Your own jaw can make lateral movements (left and right), which is useful for chewing fruits and vegetables. But your cat cannot move his lower jaw to the right. His jaw works great for biting into flesh, tearing it apart and swallowing it whole. Our dentition works great for chewing fruits and vegetables.

Carnivores have such strong and powerful stomach acids that they can digest bones. They swallow meat without even chewing it and digest it. Our own stomach acids are very weak in comparison. If you don't chew a single tiny almond or sunflower seed, what happens? You know what happens. It goes straight through, without being digested at all.

Just look at your hands. Those hands are meant for grabbing and peeling fruits. Carnivores and herbivores can only use their mouths to eat. Even omnivores like pigs, that our modern biologist would like to classify humans with, swallow fruits whole — with the peel and everything. They don't have the hands required to peel an orange. But now look at the primates — it's so amazing to see them eat because they are so similar to us. They have hands with five fingers, just like us, and use them to grab and peel fruit. They'll peel bananas and oranges just like us. Chimpanzees will even use a rock to crack open nuts. This is just one of the dozens of observations that we can make to distinguish the various categories of animals on earth and try to find where humans fit.

Modern biologists would like to believe that humans are omnivores, like the pig. That is, we are supposed to eat anything: fruits, vegetables, meat, fish, seeds, grass — *anything*. However, this is not what the great physiologists of the past century have discovered. Physiologists have classified humans as *Frugivores*. What is a frugivore? A frugivore is simply an animal that eats *mostly* fruits and vegetables, like the primates.

The Diet of the Primates

Let's take a closer look at the diet of the primates.

Gorillas — Mountain gorillas primarily eat green vegetation (95%), partly because they don't find much else in their natural surroundings. They eat rare fruits in seasons. According to Dr. George Schaller, a very serious researcher and primatologist in this field, and Dian Fossey, another great primatologist, they do not eat any animal products. In experiments conducted at the San Diego Zoo, gorillas were given the choice between fruit and greens. The results were very interesting. The gorillas in the experiment ended up eating only fruit for the duration of the three months of the experiment.

Chimpanzees — Chimpanzees eat mostly fruits, some green leaves, nuts and sometimes meat. Animal products represent less than about 5% of their diet.

Orangutans — Orangutans eat mostly fruits, some greens, and some nuts. When fruit is rare or not available, they eat more green leaves and some insects. Animal products represent a small portion of their diet. These animals enjoy a wide variety of sweet, delicious fruits, such as rambutan, wild fig and cempedak. They are especially fond of durian.

Bonobos — The bonobos are the closest animals to human beings.

They are amazingly similar to us in many ways. Bonobos are now recognized as a separate animal from the chimpanzee. Whereas chimpanzees can be of an aggressive nature, bonobos are calmer and resolve conflicts differently (namely by having sex!). Their diet is also close to our ideal diet: bonobos eat mostly fruits with a certain type of plant similar to sugar cane, as well as various greens, young shoots and buds. They apparently do not eat any nuts. They eat some insects, perhaps small fish and small animals, but they are not seen hunting like chimpanzees. Animal products represent less than 1% of their diet.

It has been difficult to get an idea of what the ideal food of humans is, based on the diets of primates, partly because these eating patterns vary greatly from one type of primate to another and even from tribe to tribe. However, we do know that they all eat a fruit-based diet, except for the gorilla, which apparently would like to differ. And they all eat greens in significant quantities. The animal products in their diets are in very small quantities.

Obviously we have similarities with them, so our natural diet should have similarities, but we are not exactly like them, so our diet cannot be exactly like theirs. Note that when chimpanzees eat meat, they can hunt down the animal with their bare hands and eat it freshly killed. Which one of my readers could do the same?

How to Learn from Animals

How to Find The Ideal Diet
Mosséri quotes another hygienist:

During the years I spent in Central America and in Cuba, I had the opportunity to observe the reaction of monkeys when offered a food they never ate before. Instinctively, they use three senses to know if the food is poisonous.

• The sense of sight
• The sense of smell

• The sense of taste

First they attentively look at the new food. If it passes this first exam of the sense of sight, they pursue their examination with their acute sense of smell. They bring their nose close to this new food and smell it intensely. If they find it has a pleasant smell, it will have passed this part of the inspection. Finally, they lick the food and taste a small piece of it. If they like the taste, they start to eat it carefully.

During this whole process, the animal acted according to the Universal Law of Natural Dietetics; that is, they found the new food to be:

• Pleasant to the sight
• Pleasant to the smell
• Pleasant to the taste

When it was consumed:

• In the raw state
• Without combinations
• Without seasonings

This law is known by all animals, who obey it… all except man.

Theofilio de la Torre
As quoted by Mosséri in *La Nourriture Idéale*

To this description by de la Torre, a natural hygienist of the 19th century, let us add that through the process of civilization, we humans have lost much of our instinct. We cannot rely on it entirely (the mistake of "instinctive eating"). Everyone, more or less, has a debased instinct. For this reason, many authors observed children in order to get clues on what would be our natural diet.

The Instinct of Children

T.C. Fry preferred to rely on the pure instinct of children to determine our natural diet. He would imagine a table filled with all sorts of foods: fruits, vegetables, living rabbits, fish, nuts, seeds, and so on, and would ask: what would a child choose? This is how he was led to believe that our natural diet was a fruitarian diet, because a child would choose fruit in preference to all other natural, raw foods.

Dr. Shelton, in the article I quoted at the beginning, also describes how Dr. Densmore, a researcher of the past century, came to further proofs that fruits and nuts are the natural foods of humans.

> He next noted that these foods need no additions, no sweeteners, no seasonings, no preparations, to appeal to the olfactory and gustatory senses of man. "If the dishes that are set before a gourmet," he said, "those that have been prepared by the most skillful chefs, and that are the product of the most elaborate inventions and preparations, were set beside a portion of the sweet fruits and nuts as produced by nature, without addition or change, every child and most men and women would consider the fruits and nuts quite equal if not superior in gustatory excellence to the most *recherché* dishes.

Let's also add that green vegetables form an important part of the diet and are appealing in their natural state, although not as much as fruits.

Determining the natural diet with this method is a complex matter. However, we can rely on our observations of biology and the knowledge accumulated during the past two hundred years by hygienists to declare that our ideal natural diet should mainly, if not entirely, be composed of *raw fruits and vegetables*, with small quantities of *nuts and seeds*. A discussion of where the other foods could fit in the diet will be found in this book.

Again, the rational approach to nutrition, one I have followed in this book, is the following:

1) **First, determine our natural diet:** What foods are we biologically designed to eat?

2) **Second, pay attention to all of the factors that can get in the way of optimal nutrition**, by securing enough sleep, engaging in physical activity, avoiding poisonous habits (drinking coffee, taking drugs, consuming alcohol, medicines, etc.)

3) **Third, eat foods as close to nature as possible.** This means eating mostly raw, unprocessed, unseasoned, whole foods.

CHAPTER 2

Fat

Our Fat Needs

Fat is often an object of diet discussions. Is fat good for you? Is it bad for you? Should we eat a low-fat diet, or only consume "good fats"? I will be giving you some guidelines about fat consumption in this chapter, since this is one of the most important concepts to understand in order to succeed on the raw-food diet (or on any diet, for that matter).

First, it should be understood that your body doesn't need fatty foods in order to store body fat. It can create its own fat from the other non-fatty foods that you consume. A natural diet of fruits and vegetables, with some nuts and seeds or avocado, provides essential fatty acids in sufficient quantities.

All unrefined plant foods, including fruits and vegetables, contain a certain percentage of fat, which is enough to meet your needs. Even green vegetables contain essential fatty acids. Even fruit contains a small quantity of fat. Adding small quantities of avocados and nuts and seeds will certainly provide all the essential fatty acids you could ever need. There is absolutely no need to add oil to the diet, as it is a fractured, over-concentrated form of fat.

Because of their complexity, fatty foods are the most difficult foods to digest. It has been shown that a drop of oil slows down digestion for two hours.

It has been shown that excessive fat consumption, from animal or plant sources, contributes to the following health problems:

- Diabetes
- Candida
- Chronic fatigue
- Lack of energy
- Hypoglycemia
- And more

The point that needs to be understood is that too much fat, even coming from natural sources such as avocados, nuts and seeds, will create health problems. The main reason why many raw-foodists fail miserably is that they end up eating a very high-fat diet without even realizing it, or while thinking it's actually a good thing because they're eating "good fats".

The reasons people end up eating a lot of fat on a raw-food diet are simple to understand.

1) *We're used to eating concentrated foods.* The standard American diet is over 45% fat by calories, while most health organizations recommend a fat intake of less than 25%. Even vegetarians and vegans eat a diet that's high in fat.

2) *Fat is a concentrated source of calories.* We're used to eating concentrated foods such as pasta, oils, butter, bread, etc. On a raw food diet, there are practically no concentrated foods other than fatty foods. Thus, people often find themselves compensating for their lack of caloric intake by eating concentrated fatty foods.

3) *The only alternative to fat is fruit.* On a raw food diet, there are basically two types of food that provide calories (energy): fruit and fat. Vegetables are so low in calories that it would be impossible to survive eating just vegetables. To get 2000 calories, which is barely enough to meet the needs of most people, you would need to eat 20 heads of lettuce! On a raw food diet,

you don't eat starchy foods (bread, pasta, etc.), which are the main sources of complex sugar in a standard diet. So the only alternative to get enough calories besides eating excessive quantities of fat is to eat a lot of fruit.

4) *We don't eat enough fruit.* The problem is easy to understand when you realize how much fruit it takes to really give you enough energy to go through the day. A banana will provide between 100 and 140 calories, depending on the size. So if you need 2000 calories, you'd need to eat 15-20 bananas a day in order to meet your caloric needs. Since people do not eat enough fruit and haven't learned to eat enough fruit, they end up compensating by eating more concentrated fatty foods, such as avocados, durian, oils, nuts and seeds.

You have to get your calories (fuel) from somewhere. Fat is a concentrated source of calories, but it also takes lots of energy to digest. We also know that excessive fat intake leads to several health problems. On the other hand, fruit is easy to digest, provides rapid energy, and is alkaline-forming. Dr. Doug Graham says it straight:

> The SAD ("Standard American Diet") is, on average, comprised of about 42% fat. Many people on this diet eat over 50%, even 60%, of their total calories as fat. They have learned to satisfy their appetite with fats. This is not what our physiology is designed to thrive on however. A diet dominated by the simple carbohydrates found in fruit more closely matches our physiological needs. But when going raw, most people continue consuming a high-fat diet. As they eat more vegetables, they get hungrier and eat even more fat to satisfy themselves. The simple carbohydrate deficit accrues with almost every meal.
>
> When prospective raw-foodists go off their raw regimen, they almost invariably

find themselves eating cooked complex
carbohydrates. Until they learn to consume
high amounts of sweet fruits to fulfill
their carbohydrate needs, they will
invariably fail in their health and raw-
food efforts.

The high-fat raw-food diet is a recipe for
failure, both in regards to health and to
staying all raw. Utilizing the high-fruit
diet is the ideal, logical and healthful
method for achieving the low-fat, high-carb
diet that every health practitioner on the
planet recommends.
              Dr. Doug Graham

Addiction to Fat?

We can see that most raw-foodists are drawn to eating excessive
quantities of fatty foods like nuts and seeds because they do not
eat enough fruit to meet their energy needs, and because they are
used to eating heavy, cooked, fatty meals. They may have problems
with the "detox" that never ends (see chapter 7). They feel tired all
the time and blame it on detoxification. At some point, they are
convinced that supplements will correct this. So are they really
thriving?

Why not take an honest look at their diet? Someone who eats five
avocados a day. A single avocado usually weighs 300 grams (of fruit
flesh), so that's 1500 grams of avocado flesh. At 18% fat, that's 270
grams of fat, the equivalent of over a cup of oil. What would be the
consequence if you were to sit down and drink those 16 tablespoons
(or 48 teaspoons) of oil?

How Much Fat is Best?

The various health organizations of the world -- the ones that have
been around for a long time, not just those that promote the latest

fad -- recommend a fat intake that is below 25%. They recommend that level because most people eat over 45% of their total calories from fat. Cutting fat intake by half is already a big deal for most people, so that's why they come up with the number of 25%.

However, most progressive health experts, those who have been around for a long time and are still promoting the same program year after year, recommend a fat intake of *around 15% or less*. Dr. Graham, a Florida-based leader of the raw-food movement, recommends 10% or *less*.

This is congruent with the latest research that has been done on a large number of people, such as the *China Study*. The China Study is the largest nutritional study ever done (see book by the same name.) It came to the conclusion that a plant-based, low fat diet is best. The total calories coming from fat in such a diet is less than 15%.

The primates all eat a low-fat diet. Recent research also shows that our ancestors also ate a low-fat diet.

How Much Fat Do You Consume?

We know that people on the Standard American Diet consume over 45% of their total calories from fat. But research done on raw-foodists also shows that most people on a raw-food diet get over 65% of their calories from fat! Some even up to 80%! Is it any wonder that people experience so many problems on this diet?

If you want to find out how much fat you really consume, you should analyze your diet with a precise tool. I guarantee that you will find that your fat intake is much higher than you imagine.

To find out how much fat you eat, go to www.fitday.com. Open an account with them (it's free), and then enter in their database the foods you ate yesterday, for example. Do not forget to mention all the oils that may have been included in your salad dressing, and other types of "hidden" fats. I guarantee that most of my readers will have a surprise when they see that their "low-fat" diet is actually quite high in fat!

It should be mentioned that tools like this can't be totally accurate, as the caloric value of produce varies according to size, degree of ripeness, quality, etc. However, it gives you a basic analysis that is sufficient for our purposes.

In Practice

Unless you are allergic to them, I do not recommend avoiding avocados and nuts. You can eat them regularly with benefit. The following guidelines will help you:

The ideal is to limit your fat consumption to less than 15% of your calories. In practice, it means:

- Eating enough fruit to meet your caloric needs (which means a lot, by most people's standards!)
- Avoid oils (this includes olive oil, flax seed oil, coconut oil, coconut butter, etc.)
- Eat no more than one half to one avocado a day (depending on caloric requirements)
- Eat no more than two ounces (60 grams) of nuts or seeds per day. Alternatively, you could have two to four tablespoons of raw nut butter
- Eat avocados or nuts on <u>separate</u> days
- Eat fat only once a day
- Don't eat fatty food every day of the week

Some More Guidelines

- *Avoid the sweet fruit and fat combination.* If you just eat an apple, it will digest quite fast and leave the stomach rapidly. But eat an avocado at the same time and digestion will be prolonged. The sweet fruit will have time to ferment and create acidity in the body. The same happens when you mix nuts with dried fruits — an abominable combination that is likely to putrefy and ferment, unless it is consumed in very small quantities, such as five almonds with five dates.

- *You can avoid fats entirely for weeks during times of hot weather,* when the body calls for water-rich foods, such as tomatoes, cucumbers, melons, peaches, etc.

CHAPTER 3

Protein

Everyone knows that we require a certain quantity of protein to stay healthy. However, as a result of propaganda, a lot of people view the daily consumption of high-protein foods like meat and dairy as very beneficial.

The greatest fear of the new vegetarian or raw-foodist is lack of protein. Vegetarians replace meat protein with tofu, cheese, beans and meat substitutes, while raw-foodists prefer nuts and seeds (which actually contain much more fat than protein).

The opinions of experts regarding our daily protein needs vary incredibly — from 25 to 200 grams a day! An average figure is one gram per kilogram of body weight.

I personally think it is inaccurate to evaluate our protein needs by weight or grams consumed. It is more accurate to evaluate this by percentage of total calories.

So, the question is, how much protein do we need?

Most people believe that we need to eat a lot of protein in order to stay healthy. At the very least, they think that vegetarians should eat concentrated protein foods such as beans, tofu, and so on. This concept that protein is a hard-to-find nutrient for a vegetarian is very far from the truth.

Here's the reality: as long as you eat *enough calories*, it is almost impossible to have a protein deficiency, even on a very limited diet.

For example, what's the period in the human lifespan within which we require the most protein due to our incredibly fast growth? It's infancy, isn't it? And what's the protein content of mother's milk, the only food a baby should consume when it needs the most protein for its own growth? Only 6%.

That's it. Nature determined that humans do not need more than 6% of total calories from protein, even during their most intensive growth phase.

That being said, let's look at the protein content of various raw foods.

Protein Content of Fruits

Banana: 4%	Papaya: 7%
Peach: 7%	Avocado: 5%
Orange: 9%	Watermelon: 7%

Average protein content of fruit: 5%

Protein Content of Vegetables

Tomatoes: 17%	Cucumber: 21%
Lettuce: 59%	Celery: 25%

Average protein content of vegetables: 20%

Protein Content of Nuts & Seeds:

Almonds: 15%	Sesame Paste (tahini): 12%
Sunflower seeds: 15%	Pumpkin seeds: 17%

Average protein content of nuts and seeds: 15%

- ***Average protein content of a low-fat raw food diet: 7-8%***
- ***Average protein content of human milk: 6%***

Some People Live on Very Small Amounts of Protein

During an expedition in the interior regions of New Guinea, the researchers Hipsley and Clements of Sidney discovered an aboriginal tribe living in the mountains of Mount Hagen whose diet consisted mainly of certain plants, 80% to 90% of their diet was sweet potatoes. The rest was composed mostly of young shoots, sugar cane, green vegetables, bananas, palm hearts and various nuts…The population, including the children and teenagers, was obviously in very good health, while accomplishing great physical work.

Professor H.A.P. Oomen... discovered that their daily consumption of protein was 9.92 grams (due to the fact that sweet potatoes only contain between 0.5 and 1.5% protein.) Meanwhile they eliminated in their fecal matter around 15 times more protein than was ingested through their diet, eating between 1.4 and 2 kilos of sweet potatoes a day. The logical conclusion was that proteins were synthesized in the body following an unknown process.

Albert Mosséri
La Nourriture Idéale

There are other cultures in which people live on root-based diets and obtain an average of less than 5% of their total calories from protein, while remaining in great health. The World Health Organization (WHO) proved that, considering the fact that the body recycles most of its protein for its own needs, 5% is more than enough. However, most vegetarians are still terrified by not getting enough protein. As soon as they feel a lack of energy, they think to themselves, "Could it be a lack of protein?"

Where do you get your protein?

As we have seen, there is plenty of protein in raw foods. Even fruits contain at least 5% of their total calories from protein. As long as you eat enough to meet your caloric needs (we'll be discussing this more later in the book), and you eat a good variety of foods, there is absolutely no need to fear any protein deficiency.

A raw-food diet of fruits and vegetables, even if it doesn't include a lot of nuts and seeds, provides about 7-10% of protein a day. This is more than what the WHO says is a safe amount. And it is more protein than contained in mother's milk.

In spite of these facts, many authors recommend eating too much protein. Excess protein is actually not healthy, just like excess fat.

There is a lot more about this topic that could be said and in this chapter I have just given you an overview. More information on protein will be found in my course, *How to End Confusion About Nutrition,* available from www.fredericpatenaude.com/ starterkit.html

CHAPTER 4

Nuts & Seeds

The Diet of Primates, or How to Know What to Eat

The first authors to write about raw-foodism and *Natural Hygiene* tried to find out what the ideal human diet was. To find an answer to this puzzle, they studied the diet of primates, declared by science to be our "closest relatives", thus hoping to find in the regimen of these hairy creatures the most appropriate menu for humans wishing to conform to the laws of Nature (with a capital N!).

But in view of the fact that the great apes were getting rare, and the costs and difficulties of travel were very high, paying them a visit in the heart of the jungle was not a practical solution. Instead, they examined the few zoological studies existing at the time.

Somewhere in those books, someone said that the primates lived on fruits, vegetables, nuts and seeds. This affirmation didn't stun our budding rawists. Aren't these foods the most pleasing to the palate when eaten in the raw state? All the rest (grains, dairy, meat, etc.) have to be seasoned and cooked to be appreciated. On the other hand, fruits, vegetables, nuts and seeds can be eaten with delight without any seasoning or cooking.

By using this reasoning, early vegetarians, natural hygienists and raw-foodists claimed everywhere that fruits, vegetables, nuts and seeds, consumed in their raw state, constitute the natural diet of humans.

But since then many things have changed that confuse the picture. We have learned that gorillas eat mostly greens, almost no fruit and no nuts or seeds. Orangutans, on the other hand, eat mostly fruit, *very few nuts* and some greens. And then there are the bonobos who eat 80% fruit and almost no nuts and seeds.

Problems From Excessive Nut Consumption

Some authors have started to question the value of nuts in the raw-food diet. They have done this not by scientific reasoning, but after noticing the problems that eating too many nuts brought, on themselves and their patients.

But there have always been those in favor of eating a lot of nuts, essentially because they are the only protein-rich foods in the raw vegetarian diet. Because protein deficiency has frightened us, we took comfort in the daily consumption of nuts, without realizing that nuts are not even concentrated in protein; they are concentrated in fat.

Herbert Shelton and other raw-foodists recommended around 100 to 120 grams of nuts a day, which is about a large handful of almonds (around 50-70 almonds). This would bring our total fat consumption for the day to about 50-60% of total calories. This is way more than what is recommended. Let's add that few people are able to digest this quantity of nuts every day. The French natural hygienist, Albert Mosséri, wrote:

```
I observed innumerable problems and
even serious accidents following such
a consumption of nuts: liver problems,
skin disorders, dizziness, fatigue,
lowering of the digestive powers, urinary
infection, pus, smelly and abundant urine,
lowered vision, myopia, sensitivity
to cold, sensitivity to sun baths and
light, spaciness, frequent gases, etc. I
```

> understood at once that Shelton, for all
> his genius and for all the admiration
> and respect I had for him for years,
> had committed in this matter a terrible
> mistake.
>   *La Nourriture Idéale*

Following the guidelines provided in chapter 2, it is possible to eat nuts without running into these problems.

In Nature

Raw-foodists like to talk about what is natural versus what is not. So what is the place of nuts in the natural diet of humans? The first thing that I realized when rethinking this was that nuts are a seasonal food. They are not fresh all year round, but only two to three months out of the year. Then I found that there was a major difference between a fresh raw nut and a dried one. Dried nuts have lost their natural water and fill you more because their fat and protein concentration is higher. But is it natural to eat nuts this way?

When I was in Spain I had the occasion to taste fresh almonds straight from the tree. It was an extremely satisfying treat — crunchy, creamy, and still watery, but with a certain fat content. I thought, "Wow, this is how we're supposed to eat nuts." In comparison, the nuts we find at the health food stores have been dried (often at a high temperature), frozen at the distributor warehouse, and stored for many months. They are no longer fresh.

Those who like to compare us to the other frugivorous animals will find it interesting to study the diet of the apes. Most of them live mainly on fruits and green leaves, eating nuts when they are in season a few months of the year. Gorillas do not eat any nuts and are the biggest and strongest of all. Orangutans seldom eat nuts, and then only when they can find them. Bonobos rarely eat nuts.

The Needs of Children and Pregnant Women

Growing children have different needs than adults. My recommendations are the following: you can include some nuts in a child's diet, first in the form of nut milks. Babies and children under three years of age should have mother's milk. This is especially important for the fist six months. Nut milks do not contain enough calcium and cannot replace mother's milk. If for some reason the mother cannot nurse, the baby should be given *animal* milk, preferably goat's milk, and ideally raw.

Children can have some nuts as long as they chew them well. They can also be given raw nut butters. It is also important that children be given enough fruit to meet their energy needs, and enough green leafy vegetables every day to insure they get all the minerals they need.

Green leafy vegetables contain an abundance of minerals. Children should have green smoothies (see appendix), salads, and blended salads.

It is beneficial to eat nuts in small quantities, depending on the individual. The maximum should be around 1-2 ounces (30-60 g), about 15-30 small almonds. Athletes and strong constitutions can have a little more. You will be able to gauge this for yourself, eventually. We don't need to eat nuts and seeds every day. Eating avocados and nuts on separate days is better.

SPECIAL BOOK BONUS: If you go to www.rawsecretsbonus. com and click on "Free Book Bonuses", I will give you additional information on how to feed young children on the raw-food diet, as well as a very interesting interview with a mother who raised extremely HEALTHY children on the raw-food diet, and reveals all of her secrets.

CHAPTER 5

Dental Health & Raw Foods

The author Zephyr describes in his book, *Instinctive Eating*, the dental problems he experienced eating a raw food diet:

> Too late for my own health, I was diagnosed with "rampant tooth decay and gum disease." Almost all of my teeth need fillings; a few need root canals and crowns! When I was twenty I had one cavity. My diagnosis is that I decimated my teeth when I naively quit hygiene — thinking, "raw foods can't hurt my teeth." I let teeth-eating bacteria and fruit sugar live in my mouth relatively undisturbed for years. By the time I was aware of them they were entrenched, and I was too poor and unmotivated to handle it.

This situation is not too uncommon. In my long years of seeking and searching, I've also made a lot of mistakes. I ate dried fruit in excess, I ate many nuts and seeds (too many!), I had lots of honey at times, I've eaten my share of dates, and on top of that, I didn't brush my teeth for a good two to three years (if not more), having read in some books that brushing teeth wasn't necessary.

I made every possible mistake one can make as a raw-foodist, and one consequence has been the dental problems I have experienced. Now almost all of the teeth in my mouth have fillings, except some of my front teeth!

Now before you panic, let me hasten to make the point that most people who do things correctly do not get problems with their teeth on a raw food diet. In fact, their teeth get better. But if you don't know what you are doing, you may end up in the same place.

Due to the misinformation that I received through reading raw-food books and listening to bad advice from many ignorant or misadvised leaders in the raw-food and Natural Hygiene movement, and also due to my own ignorance at the time, my dental health has suffered tremendously.

By carefully following the advice below, you will make sure you do not run into the same problems. If you have already experienced problems with your teeth, you will be able to reverse the situation.

The reasons why raw-foodists have problems with their teeth are the following:

1) After eating, the pH in the mouth drops to a more acid state. It takes 1-2 hours for it to go back up to an alkaline state. If you are snacking often, like most raw-foodists are, the pH in the mouth will remain acid. This is a perfect environment for bacteria to do their work and produce even more acids that will create tooth decay. But this will not occur if the following factors are not present.

2) Raw-foodists eat dried fruit and dehydrated foods. Dried fruit and dehydrated foods encourage tooth decay and gum disease. Dried fruit and dehydrated foods stick to the teeth and provide PERFECT nourishment for the acid-producing bacteria that cause tooth decay and gum disease. This includes all dried fruit, fruit bars, trail mixes, dehydrated crackers, raw "burgers", as well as nuts and seeds. The dried particles in nuts and seeds, as well as other dried foods, stick to the teeth and then are "eaten up" by the acid-producing bacteria that live in your mouth. Nuts and seeds can be eaten in moderation, as long as they are soaked, blended, or eaten

with a large quantity of green vegetables. But eaten straight out of the bag, they could cause tooth problems.

3) Raw-foodists eat too many acid foods. Eating acidic foods in excess can have a negative impact on the teeth. These include lemon juice, fruit juice, citrus fruit, unripe fruit, vinegar and other acid foods. I recommend that you limit your consumption of citrus to about 2-3 oranges per day, and instead have more non acidic fruits (bananas, papayas, pears, mangoes, etc.).

4) Constant contact with sugary foods encourages tooth decay and gum disease. If your teeth are in constant contact with sugar, even the natural sugars in the form of coconut water, honey, dried fruit, fruit juice or other sugary foods, tooth decay will occur. It is not okay to sip coconut water all day long, drink fruit juices, and snack often on sugary foods.

5) Raw food diets are often deficient in many important alkaline minerals, such as calcium and magnesium that are necessary to build strong enamel. Sufficient levels of vitamin D and phosphorus are also necessary to build strong teeth. These nutrients can be obtained in a balanced diet, such as the one described in this book. For more information on this topic, see our Green for Life Program at www.greenforlifeprogram.com. This program is only available at certain times of the year so if you'd like to participate make sure you take a moment to visit that website.

If the following measures are taken, dental decay can be prevented, and teeth can be healed up to their potential. Realize that this is the very minimum you can do to insure healthy teeth for life.

1) *Rinse your mouth with water during and after eating, especially when eating fruit and acid foods.* Water and other neutral liquids wash out acidity. Whole fresh fruit will have no negative impact on the teeth if the acids are removed

promptly by sipping water as you eat and rinsing your mouth with water after you're done eating. A better idea would be to eat celery after every fruit meal. I recommend brushing your teeth after a sweet fruit meal (bananas, persimmon, cherimoya, jackfruit, etc.) After a juicy fruit meal (melon, oranges, etc), rinsing your mouth with water seems to do the job.

2) *After eating certain high-sugar fruits that tend to leave residues on the teeth, you should floss and brush your teeth (just water and a brush is fine.)* <u>Those sweet fruits are</u>: banana, date, really ripe fig, persimmon, mango, cherimoya, durian, jackfruit, sapodilla, sugar apple, sweet sapote, mammey, etc. You can also eat greens after a meal of such fruits, but brushing your teeth is a good idea. After eating other types of juicy fruits, it is not necessary to brush your teeth, but it is still a good idea to finish the meal with greens (such as lettuce and celery), and/or swish water in your mouth. (You can also use water mixed with some Celtic sea salt, to restore alkalinity in the mouth environment.) The juicy fruits include all the following and more: citrus fruits, apples, grapes, kiwis, pineapple, berries, melons, papaya, pears, peaches, plums, litchi, etc.

3) *Avoid dried fruits and dried foods.* Dried fruit and dehydrated foods are NOT raw foods and are not health foods. Replacing the oven with a dehydrator is not a good move. Eat fresh foods, not dried foods. However, if you happen to eat some dried fruit or dehydrated foods, eat an apple or some celery afterwards, and brush your teeth as soon as possible.

4) *Throw out all toothpastes immediately, and instead, brush your teeth with Toothsoap* (available from www.fredericpatenaude. com/toothsoap.html.) According to Dr. Gerald Judd, PhD: *"Reenamelization of the teeth occurs when they are clean. All toothpastes make a barrier of glycerin on the teeth, which would require 20 rinses to get it off. A good solution for clean teeth, which I have used for 5 years, is toothsoap. All oils are washed*

off the teeth and the gums are disinfected. The bacteria are killed by the soap. The teeth are then ready for reenamelization with calcium and phosphate in the diet." I have recently made available an excellent Toothsoap with a great flavor that is glycerin-free. I highly recommend it to replace toothpastes. It is available at: www.fredericpatenaude.com/toothsoap. html. Avoid constant contact with sugar. It is okay to eat a lot of fruit, but have all of it in a few meals, rather than snacking on it throughout the day. Also, avoid sipping on fruit juice, coconut water, etc.

5) *Ensure proper nutrition.* In order to build strong, decay-resistant teeth, certain important minerals must be present in the diet. Particularly important are calcium, phosphorus and vitamin D. For more information, please consult my Green For Life Program at www.greenforlifeprogram.com

6) *Remove food particles.* It is necessary to floss, but food particles that get caught between the teeth and along the gum line must be removed. You can use dental floss, or learn to use a toothpick. It is important to do this once or twice a day.

7) *Research shows that it's more important HOW WELL you brush, rather than HOW OFTEN you brush.* A good brushing with a soft brush takes *at least* two to three minutes. Reach every corner of your teeth and do a thorough job. If you've had problems with your teeth before, brushing should be very well done and can take three minutes or more. One or two such complete brushings followed or preceded by flossing per day is enough.

WANT TO LEARN MORE? If you go to www.fredericpatenaude. com/oralhealth.html you will be able to order a special report on *How to Save Thousands of Dollars in Dentist Bills*. I will share with you an action checklist you can use to prevent AND reverse dental problems. I will also reveal more advanced tips that are not found in this book.

CHAPTER 6

Grains & Bread

The following is adapted from an article by Albert Mosséri.

We Are Not Granivores

"All true natural hygienists are opposed to grain products. These include bread, pasta, rice, flour, cookies and crackers. It seems very difficult for most people to understand this subject, because unconsciously they refuse to abandon the habit of eating bread and other grain products. 'It is the very foundation of civilization,' they say. Those who call themselves natural hygienists and still promote bread, even whole wheat, are not true hygienists. They don't understand that nature doesn't produce bread, that grains are meant to be eaten by birds, which are granivores (eaters of grains) and that humans are frugivores (eaters of fruit and green leaves).

"There are many reasons why grains are not suitable for humans. Among the most valid are those taken from the science of biology — and consequently, are the same types of arguments that vegetarians use to condemn meat eating.

"A chart of comparative anatomy reveals that humans have none of the characteristics of the carnivore. They do not have appropriate teeth to bite the prey, nor an adequate liver to neutralize all the toxins, and so on. Vegetarians can easily understand that humans are not carnivores. But what I say is that humans are not granivores either. We are not biologically designed to eat grains. For every class of animal on the planet, nature has provided certain categories of foods for them. Any deviation from that will create all sorts of problems -- disease, cancer, etc.

"A machine that is supposed to function well with a certain type of oil will not function as well with a different type of oil. It will clog up and break down. This is the major argument against grains. All other 'scientific' arguments are only in the details.

"Nature has provided a special type of food for fish, another type of food for cows and something entirely different for bears. And for us, nature provides us with our natural foods: fruits and vegetables. Nature is not chaotic. Every species eats the food it was designed to eat. If horses started eating meat and lions started grazing with the cow, it would be the end of everything!

The Gizzard

"Bread and grains, whole or not, are extremely deficient in minerals compared to fruits and greens. They are lacking in alkaline minerals such as calcium. Indeed, they are some of the most acid forming of all foods. Our physiology is not designed to handle the digestion of grains. The ptyalin enzyme in our mouth can only handle small amount of starch found in roots and some fruits.

Species that are granivores, like some types of birds, have a special organ called the gizzard. What is a gizzard? It's a sort of second stomach that permits certain types of birds to grind hard seeds in order to digest them. With this type of strong stomach, they can even pulverize little rocks in no time. In fact, they swallow rocks to help grind grain. Even metal needles swallowed by some young birds are broken into pieces and eliminated with no apparent damage.

"Have you ever seen chickens and other types of fowl eating rocks, nails and other hard and indigestible things? At that moment, you probably asked yourself, why are these animals eating these useless and harmful things? Have they gone mad? Or are they following their instinct? They are simply introducing hard things into their gizzard to help grind the hard seeds that they just ate.

"Birds and fowl have no teeth. That's why they have to swallow whole seeds. But since they need to digest them, nature provides them with a perfect grinding machine attached to their stomach. Small rocks when eaten serve as millstones.

"But humans are much different. They do not have a gizzard. They cannot grind hard seeds like grains or legumes. This is one reason these foods are not meant for us.

"Now someone will say that we can replace the gizzard with a millstone constructed by humans, and cook the grains to soften them and render them easy to chew and digest. That's what we've been doing for several thousands of years. But this does not solve the problem.

"The digestive tract of humans and of all frugivorous animals is too long for the efficient digestion of heavy starches. These foods stay there for too long and thus have a tendency to ferment. Grains are natural foods for birds and fowl, but not for humans. We are not equipped with a gizzard and other physiological designs in order to process grains properly.

"Furthermore, humans cannot eat and enjoy these foods in their natural state. They are simply not foods we are biologically meant to eat. Our natural foods are fruits and green leaves."

Here is Albert Mosséri's list of diseases caused by grains and bread, based on his decades of helping thousands of ill people back to health.

Diseases and Conditions Caused or Aggravated by Bread and Grain Consumption
by Albert Mosséri

- Common cold
- Flu
- Sinusitis
- Bronchitis
- Pneumonia
- Colitis
- Asthma
- Allergies
- Diabetes
- Arthritis
- Arteriosclerosis
- Heart attacks

CHAPTER 7

Detoxification

The great hygienist, Herbert Shelton, in his health classic, *The Science and Fine Art of Food and Nutrition*, says this about detoxification:

> Every adaptation to habits, agents and influences which are inimical to life is accomplished by changes in the tissues which are always away from the ideal. The renovating and readjusting process that must follow a reform in living is accomplished by the tearing down and casting out of these unideal tissues. New and more ideal tissues take their place. The body is renewed.
>
> This process of readjustment is not always smooth. Aches and pains, loss of weight, skin eruptions, etc., may result. Helen Densmore truly says that, "If it were true that, after many years of abuse, we could stop the wrong course of living and all the blessings of health follow immediately, it would be proof that this disobedience is not so bad after all.
>
> As she says, "With the drunkard, the curative action is recognized at once — all know that it is not the water that is making him ill, but the alcoholic poison which he had been before accustomed to. So mother, sister, sweetheart and friends with one accord appeal to him to keep up

his courage, notwithstanding his apparently
bad symptoms. How differently is the
poor dyspeptic treated when he attempts
to reform his diet. With one accord his
friends try to prevail on him to abandon
it; assure him that he is killing himself;
read him tomes of medical authorities to
show that he is impoverishing his blood by
his 'low diet' and when he returns to the
old injurious diet, just as with the dram
of spirits in the case of the drunkard, the
effect is to stop the curative action; he
feels braced up and this is taken as proof
that he was all wrong and the accumulation
of disease commences again.

These renovating crises are seldom severe
and are always followed by better health.
Persistence and determination are required
when they come. Most people, particularly
young and vigorous ones, will make the
change with very little or no discomfort.

Many of you may have heard of the concept of detoxification. When
you adopt a clean diet based on fruits and vegetables, your body
will begin to eliminate its accumulated toxins. Since their poisonous
nature is more noticeable on the way out than when they are "in
storage", you will probably feel worse for a while before you start
feeling better.

When you improve your diet, you may initially experience a fatigue
that, in fact, is just a relaxation. Your body is letting go of its toxins in
storage. This can take a few months — in most cases four to eight.
During this time it is imperative to sleep more, get plenty of rest
and avoid hard physical exercise and mental stress until the energy
starts to come back naturally. From this point forward you can start
exercising to build muscle and keep feeding yourself properly.

Certain cycles within the body will lead to periods of detoxification, tissue repair and growth, and so forth. You will discover that some days the body has lots of energy at its disposal and rebuilds damaged tissues. On other days your body goes through a phase of detox, and you experience lower levels of energy. The evolution of this process is impossible to predict for everybody, but the fact that it will happen is certain. One day, the body may decide to cleanse heavily, and that won't be pleasant. Once a certain level of health has been reached, you do not notice the cycles as much and they cause progressively less discomfort.

The Never-Ending Detoxification

Some people think that detoxification — the intense phase of purification — goes on forever. Years after changing their diet, they still talk about how they are "detoxifying". They attribute every headache or discomfort to the elimination of ancient toxins, while ignoring their present habits. I've known long-term raw-foodists who blamed their headaches on vaccines they received in their childhood!

This so-called "detox" that never ends is actually no detox at all, but is caused by eating the wrong, high-fat raw-food diet, and might also be caused by not eating enough fruits and vegetables to meet your energy needs. Usually, this detox is just another word for "This diet doesn't work."

In most cases, the real, intense detoxification is over within a few months. You will still eliminate metabolic waste for the rest of your life, but intense healing crises will occur rarely if you follow the advice in this book.

Once you stop waking up in the morning with a bad taste in your mouth, this intense period of detoxification is basically over. So it doesn't make any sense to blame continuing symptoms on past mistakes. Rather, think about what you are doing now that could be draining your energy. Here are some possible causes (in no particular order):

Possible Causes for Lack of Energy

- Lack of sleep
- Eating too many fatty foods, such as avocados, nuts and seeds
- Using oil
- A sedentary lifestyle
- Negative emotions
- Over-training
- Lack of fresh air
- Lack of sunshine
- Dehydration
- Chronic stress, loneliness and anxiety
- Bad food combinations
- Eating without hunger
- Overeating
- Use of spices, salt, and condiments
- Second-hand smoke

Each of these factors, and many more, will drain your energy and elevate your levels of internal toxemia. When you improve your diet, you become more sensitive, so your body will let you know more quickly when there's something wrong.

The True Prevention

When you feel mild symptoms such as headaches, fatigue, lack of concentration or irritation, analyze your lifestyle and diet over the last few weeks or months to determine what could be the reasons for your ills. Then eliminate the causes, and get extra rest. If necessary, fast for a few days on water. Albert Mosséri, the hygienist, sheds light on this subject:

> According to the Law of the Evolution
> of Disease, examined in my book *Put*
> *Your Health into the Hands of Nature*,

the various diseases always begin with unnoticed signs. For example, light headaches may be felt, or bad digestion, lack of appetite, fatigue, a fogged and unclear mind, pessimistic ideas, bad mood, gas, constipation, vague pains here and there, etc.

At the first signs of discomfort or poor health, the appropriate measures should be taken: rest, fasting, proper diet and the removal of the cause. The evolution of disease is thus stopped and no complications will occur.

But if we neglect this or we suppress these first premonitory signs by convenience — we don't want to stop working; or we prefer to suppress the symptoms with medicines and to keep drinking coffee, eating meat, bread, etc. — we then stop the redeeming elimination and prepare the grounds for diseases that will afflict the person in a very precise order, from acute to chronic.

This is how we can foresee the disease and detect it, without inefficient laboratory testing and analysis, and finally obviate its harmful consequences with a simple hygienic prevention. "Prevention is better than cure," and it is while taking care of the first symptoms that we can prevent every disease.

Mangez Nature, Santé Nature

It's Not Normal to Feel This Way

Even if you have no serious, life-threatening health problems to start with, after a year of eating a raw food diet (or any diet) it is not normal to still:

- Feel really tired in the afternoon, even if you've had enough sleep the night before
- Not have enough energy or desire to exercise
- Experience many ups and downs in energy levels
- Feel worse than before you started the diet (after the initial months of detox)

- Feel itchiness
- Have a strong body odor
- Have regular headaches
- Have more dental problems

If these conditions persist, take another look at your eating and living habits in light of the information presented in this book.

CHAPTER 8

The Law of Vital Accommodation

> The Law of Vital Accommodation is nature's
> wheel. The response of the vital organism
> to external stimuli is an instinctive one,
> based upon a self-preservative instinct
> which adapts itself to whatever influence it
> cannot destroy or control.
> > *Herbert Shelton*
> > *Orthobionomics*

Understanding the Law of Vital Accommodation may be one of the most important lessons in this book. It will help clarify many blind spots. This law states that when a poison is introduced into the organism on a regular basis, to a degree beyond the body's capacity to expel it, the body adapts to this invader by insulating itself from it. This is done at the expense of normal body functioning. For example, if you smoke, your body will prevent absorption of the toxic fumes by hardening the lung membranes to avoid intoxicating the body beyond a certain level of toleration.

If you take a less-than-fatal dose of poison every day, after six months you could take a more-than-fatal one and survive. The body will resist the poison by avoiding absorption at all cost. But this also means that general nutrient absorption will be diminished.

In *Orthobionomics*, Shelton wrote, "Toleration to poisons is merely a slow method of dying. Instead of seeing in the phenomena of toleration something to be sought after, it is something to seek to avoid the necessity for."

A Purer Body

When you begin a clean diet based on fruits and vegetables, you are no longer taking in a lot of popular poisons: coffee, chocolate, cigarettes, spices, food preservatives, etc. Your body rejects accumulated poisons and goes back to a more original, pure state -- like that of a child. In other words, you will be like a beginner, before he starts to take his daily dose of poison, which means that you will be much more affected, and penalized, by small doses of poisons than most people. A cup of coffee could have the same effect on you as five cups on your neighbor. You will be more affected by what you eat, especially if you go off your new diet. Shelton reiterates:

> The first smoke or the first chew of tobacco usually occasions a very powerful action against it on the part of the organism. The young man or woman is made very sick; there is headache, nausea, vomiting, loss of appetite, weakness, etc. So long as the physiological powers and instincts are undepraved and unimpaired, they instantly perceive the poisonous character of the tobacco and give the alarm to the whole system. A vigorous effort is made to destroy and eliminate it and the user is forced to throw away his tobacco. But if he continues to repeat the performance, the action against it grows less and less with each repetition, until, finally, he is able to use many times the original amount without occasioning such results. His system learns to tolerate it and adapt itself to its use as far as possible.
> *Orthobionomics*

You may think that eating a tiny bit of junk here and there might be okay: a piece of chocolate, a cup of coffee, a muffin, etc. But it will not be like the old days. Your body may violently reject the junk foods each time, and these small dietary divergences may destabilize and ruin everything in the long term. *Small, but regular deviations can vitiate our efforts, prevent the desired results and make one feel worse than before.*

This is why I recommend avoiding the yo-yo effect of going back and forth between one diet and another. Once you're ready to give up something, give it up completely. Stick to your diet as determinedly (though not fanatically) as possible.

Yet, you have to distinguish the big mistakes from the small ones. Eating some rice once in a while is without consequences, as compared to drinking coffee every day.

Poisons and Habits to Avoid

- Coffee, tea, and other caffeinated beverages.
- Alcohol
- Tobacco
- Marijuana
- Drugs (legal and illegal)
- Chocolate and cacao (cooked or raw)
- Spicy food, cayenne, black pepper, etc.
- Junk food
- Fried foods
- Products coming from a factory
- Household chemicals (including personal care products)

CHAPTER 9

How to Give Up Bad Habits

A Popular Tendency

There is a popular tendency in the health movement that strives to do everything possible in order to appeal to the largest number of people. It assumes that most people are not ready for big changes. It assumes that they need to take baby steps, gradually and smoothly changing their habits until they are ready to see the bigger picture. Furthermore, it assumes that most people are not ready to hear a radical message and will even frown upon it.

The experts in this frame of mind not only assume that people are incapable of great change, but also propose that people should only be encouraged to implement good habits, like eating more fruits and vegetables, rather then abandon bad ones, like eating meat. So, they will suggest "Eat less meat," rather than "Become a vegetarian," which would be viewed as a move too extreme by the majority. They will propose, "Eat more fruits and vegetables," but not "Eliminate grain products." They will suggest "Start juicing," but not "Stop smoking," or "Get more exercise," instead of "Stop taking medications," and so on.

This philosophy is embodied in the saying "An apple a day keeps the doctor away." It suggests that it does not matter how many bad habits you have : as soon as you implement good new habits, such as an apple a day, your health will improve. Eventually the advice devolves to "Take this supplement or drug, and it will compensate for whatever bad habits you may have."

Naturopathic books are filled with such insipid recommendations, the benefits of which are largely unproven and cost little or nothing to the readers. Here are some examples: take cold showers to have more energy (useless stimulation), take herbal teas for specific diseases (instead of looking for the cause), take juices to heal yourself (using food as medicine), etc. They prefer to do this rather than talk about the harmful effects of grains, coffee, salt, chocolate, meat and dairy products. This would discourage the reader who, presumably, does not want to change his diet but only get a cure for his problems.

A man suffering from high blood pressure goes to his doctor. He smokes cigarettes, eats fried foods, meat, salt, and bread, and consumes almost no raw fruits and vegetables. The doctor wants to prescribe pills for him, but he won't hear of it. He goes to a naturopathic doctor. In addition to recommending a few herbal teas, the naturopath tells him that he should "think about" stopping smoking, eat "more fruits and vegetables" and "less meat" The man leaves with what he came for: a few easy excuses for not radically changing his habits. *Why not also point out the culprits, instead of just hailing the saviors?*

Good Habits or Bad Habits?

You shouldn't measure your health solely by how many good habits you have, but also by how many bad ones you have. In other words, it doesn't matter so much, however healthy it may be, that you eat "lots of fruits and vegetables," that you "juice daily," and that you "work out four times a week," if you also indulge in coffee, bread and meat. Your health will be directly affected by your bad habits, no matter how many good ones you have. These bad habits create illness. You will not get rid of them, no matter how many good new habits you implement, unless you reform your lifestyle entirely.

Already I hear the voices of contention. Some people dislike this "negative" approach. Yes, it is negative. But so what? It's honest! Why not be true to facts and yourself, thereby improving your health?

I am not saying that you shouldn't use psychology and sensitivity. Even those who are ready to reform their lifestyles are rarely capable of doing so in one day. However, it's time to stop fooling ourselves thinking that by changing one or two things in your lifestyle you can improve your health.

Two Approaches

The typical advice goes like this: "You have to change your lifestyle, one piece at a time. You will slowly and gradually add more fruits and vegetables, and get more exercise and daily sunshine. Meanwhile, you will gradually reduce your consumption of junk food, meat, dairy and pasta.

The intelligent advice goes like this: "You have to change your lifestyle, one piece at a time. You have several bad habits that drain your energy and are the cause of your illness. You smoke, drink coffee, and eat meat, bread and cheese. Each of these habits has to be abandoned and replaced by good habits. However, I know it can be difficult, so I will help you do it gradually. Every week or two, or at whatever rate is comfortable for you, *get rid* of one of these habits, until your entire lifestyle has changed. At the same time, I will teach you new healthy habits that will be both fun and interesting."

The first approach rarely has success, because it disregards basic psychology. We gladly accept something to do, as long as it doesn't involve getting rid of the bad habits we love. We almost never let these go, unless we are told we absolutely have to (and even then, most people don't change.) In other words, "gradually include more fruits and vegetables and exclude junk food in the diet," will be loosely interpreted. We'll grab an apple here and there, maybe order orange juice instead of a coke, and make a handful of other little changes that will hardly make a difference.

It is easier to think about starting to juice than ceasing to drink coffee. This is basic psychology. You don't want to stop drinking coffee, because it is something you like. Starting to juice is easy. But stopping a bad habit is not. It takes work and determination. The easier way is more appealing. It's easier to "add" than to "remove", where habits are concerned. I wish it were as easy as taking a pill, biting a few apples, and/or eating some extra salad. Everyone likes to cling to bad habits (including me.) We must find courage to face reality and decide, "*Yes; we're going to make some real changes!*"

We must also consider the sources of advice and what they stand to gain. There's no money in telling people that they have to stop their bad habits in order to be healthy. There's no money in merely telling them to stop smoking. But there's plenty in selling them a nicotine patch. There's no money in telling people to stop drinking coffee and alcohol. But there is in selling them a juicer. There's no money in telling people to stop eating fried foods, bread, meat and dairy. But there is in selling them supplements.

What's Worse?

When it comes to bad habits, there are degrees of evil. Not all habits are equally damaging. Quantities and regularity also matter. Drinking two cups of coffee a day is not the same as drinking one a month.

In light of the principles exposed in the previous chapter, here are some bad habits that undermine health (roughly in order of importance).

- Use of drugs, prescribed or illicit
- Overeating
- Lack of exercise
- Indulgence in chronic stress and negative emotions
- Coffee, cigarettes, alcohol, tea, chocolate and other popular poisons
- Junk foods: fried foods, fast food, factory food, etc.

- Lack of sleep
- Eating foods that are not specific to the human race: bread, grains, meat, fish, dairy products, etc.
- Using condiments, spices, salt, etc., which hinder digestion and lead to overeating
- Poor food combining
- Lack of sunshine.

There are many more bad habits. These are just some of the most common.

Being Effective

Of course, people are a little better off eating more fruits and vegetables and getting more exercise. Sometimes, supplementation can mitigate an abominable diet and save someone from certain death by mineral and vitamin deficiency. But they won't get the desired results until they give up coffee, stop smoking and exclude bread, cheese, etc. from their diet. You will never "burn off" the effects of your poor diet, no matter how many miles you run, how many supplements you take, or how much sunshine you get. The idea is not to try to be perfect, but rather to take an honest look at your habits and reform your lifestyle gradually.

CHAPTER 10

Supplements & Super-foods

Supplements Among Vegetarians and Raw-Foodists

Supplements are as popular among vegetarians and raw-foodists as in the general population. However, the types of supplements consumed by these two groups are different. While the average supplement consumers buy cheap vitamin and mineral supplements in hopes of "correcting" their poor diet, vegetarians and raw-foodists buy expensive, exotic, quality supplements, either out of fear that their diet might be inadequate, or belief that these fancy products are the missing pieces in the puzzle on which "super health" depends.

Super-foods and many supplements are supposed to bring you exciting results. Blue-green algae, MSM, green powder, enzymes, horsetail powder, noni fruit, aloe vera juice, fruit and vegetable juice powder — the list is endless. What should we think of all these products? Can they be useful, or are they just another way for opportunists to fatten their wallets?

If someone feels great, she could only be led to buy tons of supplements out of fear of future deficiencies. She would have to be convinced that, although she may feel fine right now, many years from now she could run into big troubles because her diet is lacking in minerals, enzymes, vitamins or whatever. So, she'd rather play it safe and take the supplements.

On the other hand, a person who doesn't feel so great can be convinced much more easily. Many become vegetarians or raw-foodists in the hope of reaching superior health. They know that they have to go through a detox period — but a few years later, still not feeling the results, they start to wonder if there is something wrong with the diet itself. Of course, they are right. There is something wrong with the way they eat, but the supplement hucksters and naturopaths are planting an entirely different doubt in their minds. They will imagine that they feel poorly because their diet is lacking in whatever some supplement is "packed" with. They then proceed to spend $200 a month to buy supplements and other exotic articles. They might feel a little better, but where's the "Paradise-Health?"

Why would raw-foodists, who are supposed to have found the most natural diet there is, need supplements? The supplements industry offers simple, yet convincing reasons, such as: the soil is of a poor quality; the fruits and vegetables we buy do not contain enough vitamins and minerals, or the fruit is picked too early and has not reached maturity; and if we do not supplement, we will run into trouble.

The nutrition researcher Dr. Joel Fuhrman, having gone through a lot of the research available, says in his book *Eat To Live*:

> Contrary to many of the horror stories you hear, our soil is not depleted of nutrients. California, Washington, Oregon, Texas, Florida and other states still have rich, fertile land that produces most of our fruits, vegetables, beans, nuts, and seeds. America provides some of the most nutrient-rich produce in the world.
>
> Our government publishes nutritional analyses of foods. It takes food from a variety of supermarkets across the country, analyses it, and publishes the results. Contrary to the claims of many health-food and supplement enthusiasts, the produce

```
grown in this country is nutrient-rich and
high in trace minerals, especially beans,
nuts, seeds, fruits and vegetables.
```

It is my belief, as well, that soil depletion is the not the biggest problem we face. Our main problem is a lack of assimilation due to improper food choices.

What Causes Deficiencies

If you are suffering from a deficiency, it may be caused by impaired assimilation, not by a lack of nutrients in foods. Mosséri explains:

```
Let's take the case of anemia. There is an
iron deficiency in a patient. The analysis
shows it. But when we scrutinize the
patient's menu, we find in most cases that
there isn't a lack of iron! In many cases,
there is plenty of iron in the diet. In
fact, in pernicious anemia, there is an
excess of iron-based pigments in all the
internal organs. Hunter discovered that,
even in fatal cases, a great quantity of
iron leached from the blood could be found
in the spleen. This shows that there is
more iron than is needed in the bodies of
anemic people; it's just not being used.

Another proof that anemia is not caused by
a lack of iron in the diet is that this
disease regresses during fasting, when no
food is eaten and no iron is provided to
the body through the diet. During a short
fast, we notice a marked increase in the
red blood cell count. This shows that
there are iron reserves in the body, but
that, for some reasons, they are not used.
This proves that iron found in foods and
iron accumulated in the tissues has not
been appropriated, because assimilation
```

is failing. This is called a faulty
metabolism.

So we are not witnessing in these cases
an iron deficiency in the menu, but a lack
of iron absorption. This deficiency is not
of an immediate dietary origin, but could
be after a long time. After a seven-day
fast, the red blood cell count increases
noticeably. But if the fast is longer —
very long — we will be sure to witness a
lowering of the red blood cells count —
and of many other elements — because the
reserves will be used up at some point.
This is why no analysis should be done for
many months after breaking a fast.

In addition, when iron is prescribed in a
food form, such as in artichoke extracts,
no results are obtained either. What do we
gain by feeding anemic people with iron-
rich foods, when they already possess in
their tissues abundant iron reserves,
unused because they cannot be assimilated?
>   *Albert Mosséri*
>   *Mangez Nature Santé Nature*

As an example: nearly everyone drinks milk as a calcium
supplement, yet many end up suffering from osteoporosis anyway.
No matter how much calcium they take, they will not get better until
they discard the various causes that prevent calcium absorption
or leach calcium from the body. These include: caffeine, excessive
quantities of protein in the diet, cigarette smoking, inadequate
vitamin D, salt intake (including sea salt) and certain medications.

I do not recommend routine supplementation. I believe
supplements can also cause problems, instead of solving them.
I recommend instead eating a nutritious diet that provides you
with all the vitamins and minerals that you need, instead of
supplementing.

There are some exceptions to this. As you will see at the end of this chapter, vitamin B12 can be an issue. In other cases, other supplements may be required.

Enzymes in Raw Foods

There have been some hype and misinformation spread in the raw-food movement on the topic of enzymes. I personally don't think that the raw food diet gives any certain results because of enzymes. I think it's more because the diet excludes foods that are not specific to human beings (grains, beans, meat, dairy and others), leaving only fruits, vegetables, nuts and seeds. In my opinion, cooking is not problematic because it destroys the enzymes, but mainly because it creates new molecules, possibly toxic, by exposing fats, proteins and carbohydrates to high temperatures.

Here's an example of the hype. We are told to eat papayas because of enzymes. There are plenty of enzymes in green, unripe papayas. But as the fruit ripens, the enzymes convert all that starch into simple sugar. When the fruit is fully ripe, the enzymes are almost all gone! Strange? No, the enzymes are only needed by the fruit to transform complex substances (starch) into simple substances (sugar). They are not needed for digestion because the ripe fruit is fully digestible, without any of them, if any at all.

One of my correspondents wrote:

```
1)   Enzymes are biological catalysts and
the definition of a catalyst is that it is
something that alters/speeds up a reaction
without being used up in the process.
So, by definition, we cannot "run out of
enzymes." Even if we could:

2)   Enzymes are proteins and are made up
of the same amino acids as other proteins
needed in the body. Thus, if more are
```

needed, more can easily be made from the same materials as other body parts! Our raw plant foods actually go to make up enzymes!

3) Enzymes are specific — they catalyze one reaction and one reaction only. That means that plant enzymes are there to deal with reactions connected with the plant's life and not to help humans digest food. Look at the speed at which fruit ripens and then decays. It takes days, if not weeks! But human digestion of fruit takes only hours. How can the same enzyme suddenly do that? Simply, it can't. Also, enzymes being specific, human metabolic enzymes cannot logically be used as digestive enzymes. They are there only to catalyze the metabolic reaction.

In my opinion, the food enzyme theory and its wide following is one of the major things against more mainstream acceptance of raw foodism as a whole. It's blatantly wrong and gives those who insist on it a bad name. If the raw and natural food movement wishes to gain wider credibility, it has to be more credible."
      Elizabeth, UK

Raw-foodists believe that they spare their enzyme "reserves" by eating all raw. But many foods contained in a typical raw food diet not only contain few enzymes, but also use up the body's own digestive enzymes (such as dried nuts and seeds, all oils (even cold-pressed), tahini and nut butters.) Even sprouting does not entirely destroy the enzyme-inhibitors contained in beans and grains. They may contain a lot of enzymes, but those are difficult to digest due to the presence of these enzyme inhibitors (toxins that prevent the seed from sprouting) and raw starch.

There are many raw-foodists who take enzyme supplements.

According to them, the foods we consume, even if they are raw, do not contain enough enzymes, because they are picked mostly unripe and are sold weeks or months later. They are not fresh. Furthermore, they say, modern humans practice wrong living and eating habits, and do not produce enough powerful digestive enzymes anymore.

So what should we think of enzyme supplements in a raw food diet? Are they needed, or are they just another fad? I think that instead of worrying about enzymes, it is better to pay attention to your digestion first. If you don't feel or hear your organs, have no digestive pains and almost no gas, if your elimination is good, without bad odors or need for toilet paper, then your digestion — the purpose of dietary enzymes, anyway — is fine. Why worry about enzymes? The enzymes in foods will not digest them for you. You can eat an enzyme-rich, wrongly-combined meal and digest it poorly. The results will be fermentation (leading to lots of gas) and drained energy.

In some cases, supplemental enzymes may provide a useful aid, when the digestive powers have been compromised.

Vitamin B12

Vitamin B12 is essential for health, and it is not usually found in a strict vegan diet. Symptoms of B12 deficiency can include numbness in the hands and feet, unsteadiness and poor muscular coordination, and even cognitive deficits such as confusion, mental slowness and memory problems.

Normally, vitamin B12 is made in the intestinal flora with the help of beneficial bacteria. So the most important thing is to make sure you do not destroy your intestinal flora with the following (in order of importance.)

1) The use of antibiotics
2) Many prescription drugs

3) Many popular herbal remedies that contain caffeine and multiple toxic substances.
4) Herbal intestinal cleanses
5) Repeated colonics
6) Overeating, which causes food to ferment and produce an array of poisons and acids that will impair the intestinal flora
7) The regular use of frozen food
8) Coffee, tea and other stimulants
9) An excess of acid fruits

If you believe that you may have partly destroyed your intestinal flora (the use of antibiotics is the main culprit), you may have reason to worry about a vitamin B12 deficiency. In his article, *Vitamin B12 Recommendations for Total-Vegetarians*, Dr. Alan Goldhamer comments:

Upon reflection, we should note that in a more primitive setting, human beings almost certainly would have obtained an abundance of vitamin B12 from the bacterial "contamination" of unwashed fresh fruits and vegetables, regardless of their intake of animal products. Human vitamin B12 deficiency is very unlikely to occur in such a setting. Only very small amounts of dietary vitamin B12 are needed because our bodies do a fabulous job of recycling this essential nutrient. A person living in the ancestral environment regularly would have consumed fresh fruits and vegetables that were not consistently, fastidiously cleaned, as we routinely do today. Our current unusual degree of hygiene is useful for combating many health threats — but may leave long-term, strict vegans vulnerable to the potential problem of vitamin B12 deficiency.

Dr. Goldhamer continues, "Although most people associate vitamin

B12 deficiency with vegan diets, the majority of cases occur among people who regularly consume animal products." I have heard the same thing from several doctors and naturopaths who have had experience with B12-deficient individuals. They are mostly meat eaters. It proves that a lack of B12 in the diet is not the main cause of this deficiency, since animal products contain this vitamin. A lack of absorption, coupled with damaged intestinal flora, is the culprit.

The most important things to do to avoid B12 deficiency, in order of importance are:

1) Avoid everything that destroys intestinal flora.
2) Include a sub-lingual, B12 supplement.

Including a B12 supplement in the diet will make sure you avoid the specter of a possible deficiency. It is an "insurance policy" that most vegan experts recommend, and that I also recommend.

To close, I will share a few thoughts that come to mind when I think about supplements, in no particular order:

- My experience with many of these products is that they are an absolute waste of money.

- If soil is depleted, and the food grown in it is deficient, so is the food used by supplement manufacturers.

- These super-foods may contain tons of minerals per gram, but it would still take cups of the stuff to really make a difference. Simply look at the labels and do the math.

- The effect people get from supplements is often a drug effect. For example, dandelion greens contain a toxic substance that we can easily detect by its bitter taste. That means that you could eat a few leaves but not many more. Your body will let you know when you've eaten too many. But if you juice it and force yourself to drink it down, you may feel a "buzz", which is nothing more than a toxic overload — in essence, a drugging effect. The same goes for hot peppers. If you eat several fresh hot peppers, you may feel a "buzz" due to the toxic substance capsaicin, found in them.

- Supplements are an easy way to feel better about your diet without changing anything.

Some fanatical supplement users may present arguments that may seem hard to refute, but their claims are rarely based on solid facts. I think it is better to spend your money on whole, organic food rather than on supplements whose benefits are largely unproven.

FREE BOOK BONUS: If you are wondering about the latest supplement or whether you should take a particular product or not, make sure you subscribe to my online newsletter "Pure Health & Nutrition", where I discuss these topics in more details. If you go to www.rawsecretsbonus.com and click on "Free Book Bonuses", I will give you a free subscription to my newsletter "Pure Health & Nutrition" (A $97 value).

THE RAW SECRETS .... *Hunger*

CHAPTER 11

Hunger

```
When an individual has learned to live
instinctively in every particular and eats
only when genuinely hungry instead of for
pleasure or out of fear of offending a host
or hostess, then he or she is on the road
to a state of superior health unmatched in
modern times.
          Virginia Vetrano, MD
```

Hunger is a lost mechanism, a forgotten sensation if you will. Most people eat without hunger or don't know what hunger is. Learning to eat when hungry and listening to your body may be the most difficult part of natural eating.

I could go on, but I wish to turn this section over to a classic text by Albert Mosséri. Only a few hygienists talk about hunger. You rarely hear anyone talk about it anywhere else. But this principle, one of the most difficult to follow, because of our ill conditioning and bad eating habits, is of prime importance.

The Pleasures of Hunger

"Popular and medical opinion holds hunger to be a painful and unbearable sensation. We hear about the pangs of hunger. 'I suffered from hunger,' some people will tell you! But hunger is a manifestation of the normal functions of the body and all normal functions of the body bring pleasure. Urination, sleep, sex: these are all pleasurable functions.

"Why, then, talk about the sufferings of hunger — its pains? It is true that certain individuals experience some discomforts — but those are signs of elimination and detoxification. The person who stops smoking or drinking coffee experiences similar discomforts and similar pains coming from detoxification. These inconveniences should not lead to eating, smoking or drinking coffee.

True and False Hunger

"I wish to make the distinction between true and false hunger.

"False hunger disappears quickly, reappears again and disappears again. On the other hand, true hunger persists and becomes stronger. So, to distinguish them, we only have to wait for one hour or maybe little more. At the beginning, hunger will be weak. But the more we wait, the more strong true hunger will be.

"Appetite," writes Shelton, "is a counterfeit hunger, a creature of habit and cultivation and may be due to any one of a number of things; such as the habitual meal time; the sight, taste, or smell of food; condiments and seasoning; or even the thought of food."

"But this is not true hunger. Appetite is a false hunger."

"True hunger is not accompanied by any symptoms. There are no headaches or any discomforts. Ideas are clear, the mind lucid; we are optimistic, happy, tranquil and serene. True hunger can manifest itself spontaneously at any time of the day but not during the night. During the night, the muscles, including the stomach, relax. The stomach is not ready to handle food during the night, when at rest. However, if we feel true hunger before midnight, then a few leaves of lettuce should calm it and ensure a good night sleep."

"Fletcher said that, "in true hunger, 'water runs in the mouth." But according to me, we need to wait one hour. True hunger persists, whereas false hunger, with all its morbid and deceptive symptoms, disappears.

Contracted or Dilated Throat

"Most professional Hygienists attribute the main role in the manifestation of hunger to the glands of the throat and the mouth. Shelton attributes this active, main role to the nerves. In fact, the nerves are really what command this sensation of emptiness and dilation in the esophagus and the throat.

"It is why during moments of fatigue, worry, anger and other negative feelings, even if food is needed, the body will not signal for it or manifest hunger. The nerves will keep the throat and esophagus contracted. When conditions are again favorable, hunger manifests itself in the dilation of the throat and esophagus.

A Pleasant Sensation

"True hunger is always a pleasant sensation, even if it is urgent. A hole in the stomach, a feeling of emptiness accompanied by rhythmical contractions, a sensation of relaxation that climbs from the stomach to the throat spanning the esophagus — all these symptoms are pleasant. On the other hand, in cases of malnutrition and lack of reserves, the person can experience a diffuse hunger, the incapacity to work and to concentrate. These sensations disappear quickly within a few weeks, as the reserves are filled up. The person will then feel hunger, but his mind will be alert, vivid and lucid and his mood, optimistic and serene.

False Hunger: Like a Drug

"All the morbid symptoms of false hunger that I describe strikingly resemble the symptoms of withdrawal manifested in the smoker, the tea or coffee drinker and the drug addict when they stop taking their poison. These withdrawal symptoms are those of false hunger — they are elimination symptoms.

"It is obvious that if, during detoxification, a drug addict or a smoker takes his poison again, the unpleasant detoxification symptoms stop. But we should never stop detoxification, whether it stems from drug, alcohol, coffee, or unhealthy foods. 'The morbid symptoms of false hunger,' writes Shelton, 'are identical to those felt by drug users when they are deprived of their habitual drug.'

"Of course, the symptoms of addiction to drugs are much stronger, but addiction to food and the habit of fixed meal times end up in food intoxication and gluttony. They produce their own symptoms that we mistake for hunger.

"In his book *Perfect Health*, Haskell said that he, '…had asked thousands of people, including doctors, to describe the sensation of natural hunger. In their response, he noted the following symptoms: fainting, sensation of emptiness in the stomach, pains, etc. But all these sensation are those of appetite and not of hunger. They come from an incorrect way of eating.'

Appetite and Hunger

"Shelton compares the appetite to the desire for nicotine, alcohol, coffee, tea, and chocolate. 'No one could ever be hungry for these poisonous substances," he writes. "In fact, they serve no physiological need and are thus always harmful. No physiological demand for these substances can ever occur.'

"It happens sometimes that appetite is accompanied by various sensations of discomfort, sensations of weakness, depression, stomach gnawing, rumblings in the stomach, nausea, headaches and other morbid sensations. Shelton, again: 'According to Dr. Claunch, true hunger can be distinguished from appetite in the following manner: 'When you are hungry and you feel well, it is true hunger. But when you are apparently hungry and you feel unwell, it is false hunger.'

"I will however make an exception to this rule when the person feels faint. At the beginning of dietary change, digestion is weak, the cells are screaming for nourishment, and hunger becomes frequent and imperative.

"Some people faint and should eat quickly at these moments. After that, with the improvement of the digestive power, the reserves will be more substantial — hunger will be felt less often and will be easier to bear. With the diet of denatured and cooked foods, one digests only 20% and the rest exits in the stools the next day. However, with the new, healthy diet, composed of living foods, one digests 90% and the stools are in small quantities, well formed and odorless. So the change from one state to another creates an urgent call for food, until the digestive power improves. This hunger is a symptom of undernourishment.

"Dr. Claunch makes another useful distinction, 'When a sick person skips a habitual meal, he gets weak before feeling hunger. But when a healthy person skips a habitual meal, he feels hunger before getting weak.'

"Hunger is a sacred principle in our lives — a principle to respect at all times. Those who tell you to smell the foods to make your choice ignore hunger and are seeking appetite! The most common and worst mistake is to fill up our stomach because it's mealtime, or because the doctor told us to, or as a social distraction to please our host and guests.

A Natural Demand

"When we eat without experiencing a natural demand, we don't benefit, or we benefit very little, from what we eat. It is exactly like those who practice deep and forced breathing without any need, or those who drink without being thirsty. 'This way of eating,' writes Shelton, 'transforms the body into a fertilizer factory.'

"True hunger represents a natural demand, and furthermore, it indicates that food will be effectively assimilated by the body. On the other hand, when we smell foods before choosing a tempting one, we are looking to increase appetite. We only digest a part of what we ingest.

What Hunger is Not

"Shelton writes, "Let's see what it is not, before trying to find what it is. Think about thirst. Is it a pain? Is it a feeling of dizziness? Of passing out? It is none of this. Thirst is felt in the mouth and in the throat, and we feel a conscious desire to drink water. We never mistake a headache for thirst, because we know thirst very well. It is the same for genuine hunger. We feel a genuine desire to eat. We are at ease without pain or discomforts. The saliva runs abundantly in the mouth and often we desire a particular food.""

"Some fasting patients feel acute stomach pains that may last for a week. It is not hunger. Those that feel this are dyspeptics, nervous and anxious individuals, ulcer sufferers and those who suffer from gastritis because of unhealthy foods and medicines.""

"Certain temporary pains are due to the spasmodic contractions of the stomach and intestines, coming from the psychological or emotional disturbance of the sympathetic, abdominal nerve that controls this region of the body.

When We Faint

"According to Dr. Doods, the sensation of fainting, in certain cases, does not come from a lack of food, but rather from the absence of a habitual stimulant. But this could be objected to. In fact, this sensation should not be ignored or taken lightly. The subjects suffer from severe undernourishment because they digest only 10% of what they eat. We cannot prolong this state without risk. These persons must be fed appropriately, in small quantities at a time, with repeated small meals, in favorable conditions of rest (before and after every meal) and in the absence of all disturbances, psychological, emotional or otherwise. Shelton also mentions the sensation of fainting among the sensations of false hunger, but I consider this to be an acute symptom of undernourishment and genuine hunger.

"Let's examine more closely this sensation of fainting, an issue of gravity. When this happens, the person should eat, because the body is signaling for food, and lie down a little while. After some weeks this type of hunger disappears, to be replaced by a non-urgent hunger when the reserves are restored.

"Thus, those that feel this fainting sensation for having missed a single meal should be fed in this manner. I have encountered many similar cases of people who have consciously ignored this sensation of hunger. They kept on not eating and ended up with an uncontrollable overeating that resulted in death by undernourishment. In this state, large meals are not properly digested. They pass in the stools and exacerbate this state of undernourishment. They can lead to death by inanition. What is required in these extreme conditions are many small meals, under the control of an energetic supervisor who will not let the person gorge himself to death, but will allow him to eat just enough to calm his hunger.

When We Feel Weak

"We must not mistake this faint sensation for weakness. In this case, we feel no strength and are incapable of concentrating or making any physical effort. This is due to toxemia. The overloaded liver takes up all the blood and energy, which deprives the muscles. In these moments, one should abstain from eating, lie down and postpone the meal. The strength will come back quickly, along with mental clarity.

"However, when a person faints — a feeling of emptiness inside, a state close to passing out, a diffuse hunger that goes from the stomach and climbs up to the throat and mouth — the person should eat a little bit and then rest or take a nap. These persons can carry a few dates with them, just in case.

"Weakness, on the other hand, is not a symptom of hunger, but one of poisoning. It calls not for a cup of coffee, a cigarette or food — as is the habit of most people — but a period of rest lying down. Some people will object that in normal life, we don't always have the occasion to lie down when we are tired and that a cigarette or a cup of coffee "wakes you up," enabling you to pursue your activities. I always reply that this happens to the detriment of one's health and that, sooner or later, one will suffer the consequences. There is always a bill to pay.

The Smell of Foods and Condiments

"Contrary to what is practiced by the Instinctos (those who follow instinctotherapy), true hunger cannot be aroused by the smell, taste, or even the thought of a food. These instinctos, who sniff foods before eating them, are not hungry, but are only looking for appetite and desire. When we are truly hungry, we are not so picky in our food choices.

"On the other hand, true hunger is not stimulated by condiments, spices and salt. These substances are poisons. The saliva that pours over salt does not contain digestive juices, but water to dilute the poison and render it less corrosive to the tissues.

"When we feel true hunger, we are satisfied by simple food of any type in the natural state — without any seasoning or preparation. When we feel true hunger, we generally don't have a preference for a particular food that our sense of smell is instinctively supposed to locate and pick out. *Hunger is the best sauce.*

"However, in false hunger, one is looking for desire and appetite. One is difficult and picky.

Variety Excites Appetite

"It is known that appetite, desire and false hunger can be stimulated by variety. When we no longer want to eat a food we are full of, we can excite the appetite by changing to another food. This is why variety leads to gluttony.

"Do we have to limit ourselves to only one kind of food per meal? Maybe. Anyhow, we should not multiply the number of foods — two to three types of fruit are better than five or six. 'How many people are still hungry when it is time for dessert?' asks Shelton. 'But even so, very few refuse this dessert!'

How Many Meals a Day?

"I am often asked how many meals we should eat each day, one, two or three? It depends on your hunger. There is no sacred number. If you eat small meals, like vegetarian animals, you will need to eat three, four or even five meals a day. But if you eat large meals, like carnivores, then one or two meals will suffice.

Simple Foods

"In my opinion, any food can satisfy true hunger. On the other hand, in false hunger the person is only satisfied in the capricious choice of a particular food, according to his smell or his taste. This is why the practice of smelling foods one at a time before making a choice reflects false hunger."

Notes by Frederic

The best way to cultivate hunger is to engage in vigorous exercise on a daily basis. In fact, it is the *only* thing that will really awaken this forgotten sensation of hunger.

As an experiment to understand hunger, wait an hour before eating the next time you think you are hungry. If it is true hunger, your pleasure when eating will be even greater and you will not be able to ingest large quantities of foods because the stomach will not be distended from previous meals.

When you are truly hungry, any food can satisfy you, but sometimes we desire one category of food in particular — fruit or vegetable. When you are truly hungry, a simple apple or a head of lettuce will be a delight. It is through true hunger that eating simple, unseasoned food becomes natural and easy.

To start the practice of eating with hunger, begin with the morning meal. Earn your meal with exercise.

If you eat before going to sleep, you are not likely to sleep well, because the digestion of food will interfere with sleep. If that happens, the next day true hunger may not manifest itself before 3-4 p.m. So avoid eating or drinking three hours before going to bed.

Signs of True Hunger

- The stomach "pulls"
- The mouth salivates
- The mind is optimistic, clear, and happy
- There is a pleasant sensation in the throat
- It persists when ignored

Signs of False Hunger

- Dry mouth, coated tongue, and bad breath
- Headaches
- Rumblings in the stomach
- The mind is spacey, unclear, the spirit pessimistic
- Stomach cramps and pains, nausea
- Disappears when ignored

CHAPTER 12

Sleep

```
The mode of living in this age produces
such a waste of power and such a sense
of weariness that only the limited few
ever know the supreme delights and the
enviable luxury of power in reserve.
They keep up their semblance of vigor
by means of stimulation and seldom take
sufficient time to re-charge their vital or
nervous batteries. Nights are turned into
day, while mental and nervous poise is
exceedingly rare. All poison habits, all
excesses, the indulgence of any or all the
passions constitute distinct drains upon
the vital resources and are sources of
diminished vitality, crippled usefulness
and shortened life. Modern life presents
us with an almost unlimited variety of
means of stimulation, excitement, thrills
and dissipation chiefly originating in the
clever but perverted ingenuity of those who
reap financial rewards from these things.
          Herbert Shelton
          Orthobionomics
```

Sleep and Diet

You may have heard that raw-foodists only need to sleep five to six hours per day. I have met people who told me they only needed three to four hours of sleep a day. I even met one man who said he slept two hours a day. Impressed by this, I tried everything to be able to sleep less: juice fasting, fruit diets, etc. But I still needed my seven to nine hours of sleep.

Although it is true that the need for sleep is affected by diet, the amount of sleep required may not be the same from one person to another. You will notice that on a raw-food diet you will need less sleep, on average about 1-2 hours less.

However, if you follow my recommendations, you will also want to increase your level of fitness by exercising more. For this, you will need more sleep to recover. Usually, for every hour of physical activity, you need about an extra hour of sleep. Keep in mind that a fit person will be much more productive and energetic during the waking hours than a sedentary person.

The best advice I can give you about sleep is get as much of it as you can! And if you are trying to overcome a health challenge, the more the better.

An observation of nature will show us that animals love to rest and sleep. They get as much sleep as they wish, which, of course, depends on the species. Also, notice that young animals need more sleep than mature ones. The same holds true for humans. The younger you are, the more you need to sleep. It is also good for the elderly to get plenty of sleep. (Surveys show that most of older people do not get the amount of sleep they truly need.) Intense physical activity and training also increases your sleep needs.

The Importance of Sleep

Sleep and rest are essential to recharge your nervous energy. Your physical, emotional and mental balance depends on the quality and the quantity of your sleep. Work and play are great, but they also put demands on the body, dissipate your energy and produce metabolic waste (toxins). Rest is the only thing that recharges these "batteries" and allows for the proper elimination of metabolic waste (toxins).

It may be true that the healthier you are, the less rest and sleep you need. But since we live in such a polluted modern world, we probably would be better off securing more rest. Those with health challenges must get the maximum amount of rest, while avoiding mental and physical exertion, if they are to heal.

```
If invalids are to be restored to good
health, if strength and vigor are to take
the place of debility and weakness, we must
save life, by saving power. The conditions
of recovery are conditions of conservation
and recuperation. This principle applies to
every organ and function of the body. Rest
for each organ is as imperative as rest for
the whole body. The heart requires rest
as much as do the muscles and the arms.
The stomach must have rest the same as the
eyes. The glands of the body have the same
need for rest as does the brain. Rest, by
reducing activity, is the first requisite of
recovery.
            Herbert Shelton
            Orthobionomics
```

A bad piece of advice commonly given to chronically sick people is to get tons of exercise. The further depletion of energy caused by exercising, when they should be resting, makes their recovery difficult. There is no danger in stopping all physical exercise and getting as much rest as possible for a few months. It is also my advice to those changing to a raw food diet to get as much rest and sleep as possible, to temporarily suspend all hard, physical work, and to let your body heal. After a few months, the weight will start to come back, and then you can exercise again to build up strength.

Advice for Better Sleep

Try to sleep at regular hours. Wake up early and go to bed early. I know, you have heard this before. In a world of workaholics and party-junkies, going to bed early and at regular hours may sound boring. However, it's also the most natural thing to do and will bring you the best health. It is not part of our natural cycle to go to bed at 3 a.m. and wake up at noon. It is not part of our natural cycle to go to bed one day at 9 p.m. and the next at 1 a.m. That affects you, more than you can imagine.

An old saying is, "The hours before midnight count for double." We may have invented electric bulbs, but night is still meant for sleeping and daytime for waking.

If you have trouble sleeping, several things may be causing it. Any food or drink that contains caffeine, especially if you eat a raw food diet, will disturb your sleep. A few years ago, I drank herbal teas and green tea daily. I had read somewhere that the caffeine content in green tea was negligible. I couldn't fall asleep before 3 a.m., and it took me months to make the connection.

Other items that disturb sleep are: garlic, spices, onions, condiments and the habit of eating late at night. Your evening meal should be fairly simple, light and properly combined. Also, avoid eating sweet fruit late in the evening. The sugar and acids in fruit may prevent you from falling asleep, and they may also disturb your sleep. I recommend not eating or drinking three hours before going to sleep. Otherwise, your sleep will be disturbed by digestion, which will manifest as disturbing dreams and nightmares. What you eat before going to sleep greatly influences how you feel the next day.

If you are truly hungry before midnight, a few bites of raw vegetables, or an apple, should be enough. But avoid heavy fruits and fats. Otherwise, you may wake up tired the next day.

CHAPTER 13

Water

Water Needs

On a diet of raw fruits and vegetables with small quantities of fat, and without salt or spices, one needs little water to drink. This is because juicy fruits and vegetables contain all or most of the water the body needs. The recommendation to drink eight glasses of water a day is for those eating a grain-based, mostly cooked diet (bread, meat, cheese and starches) that is low in water, high in salt, fat and protein. However, additional water may be needed under many circumstances, even on a fruits and vegetables diet.

Your water needs increase when you exercise, in times of warm weather, and under many other circumstances. When a healthy person is well hydrated, the urination frequency is between 8 to 10 times per day. If you urinate less than 6 times per day, you are dehydrated and you need to drink more water.

When eating more dense fruits, like bananas and durian, you are well advised to drink water before the meal or to blend those fruits with water. Eating enough celery and vegetable matter will also help you stay well hydrated.

Certain fruits, like watermelon, contain a lot of water, but they also contain a sugar that enters the bloodstream really fast. The excess sugar is rejected in the urine with lots of water. Therefore, the water contained in watermelon is not even enough to handle the sugar in it (for most people.) That is why if you go on a watermelon diet you can feel dehydrated — which sounds unbelievable, but it happens. The key to watermelon is to drink some water before or after eating it. Personally, I do not eat watermelon very often.

The best waters to use are reverse-osmosis, or filtered water. In America, I would avoid drinking tap water anywhere, but in some other countries, it is permissible.

Unnatural Thirst

You may feel unnatural thirst if you eat foods that are poorly combined, eat too many nuts, seeds or avocados, eat dried fruit or eat something with salt or cheese. You can thus monitor your digestion with the thirst factor. If you feel unnatural thirst often, it means you are doing something wrong.

You may also feel unnatural thirst if you overeat sweet fruit. Eating too much sugar (more than your body needs) will cause the body to reject the excess in urine with water — leading to a dry mouth.

Unnatural thirst is an unpleasant sensation. It is one of dryness in the mouth and may be accompanied by slight dizziness. Natural thirst, in contrast, is a pleasant sensation, like natural hunger. It manifests itself as a strong, slightly exciting desire for water.

When to Drink

Water is important during transition. The body dilutes toxins and carries them out with it. Drink as much as a liter upon rising from sleep and enough throughout the day to prevent a dry mouth. Later you will find that your need and desire for additional water will decrease.

There are times when drinking water is crucial. One is during a fast, when no other food is taken. When experiencing a detoxification crisis, it is good to drink an adequate amount of water to help flush the toxins out. If you exercise a lot, you need to drink additional water, even on a fruit and vegetable diet — as much as a gallon a day. You will eventually get to know exactly how much water you need to perform your best.

CHAPTER 14

Raw-Food Recipes

Combo-Abombos

R.C. Dini, author of the infamous book *Raw Courage World*, coined the term "combo-abombo." A *combo-abombo* is a combination that is an abomination. In other words, it is a poorly combined recipe.

The raw-food cuisine is supposed to be the healthiest cuisine ever, because only raw and living ingredients are used. Juliano, the famous raw chef, says in his book, "I believe eating Raw is the healthiest and most harmonious way for us and the planet. However, I am offering you a wealth of suggestions so you can balance whatever lifestyle you choose with delicious, superior, gourmet food that enriches your body, mind and soul." (Raw: The Uncook Book, page VII)

To avoid the pitfall of cooked food, raw-foodists have created an array of raw recipes that resemble their favorite cooked dishes. You would think that these raw-food recipes are healthier than their cooked inspirations. Unfortunately, this is often not the case. Not able to rely upon the filling quality of cooked carbohydrates, raw chefs rely upon fatty foods (nuts, seeds, avocados, oils, etc.) in order to make their recipes rich and tasty. In addition to that, these recipes are often loaded with salt (either in the form of sea salt, seaweed, soy sauce, miso, or other salty seasoning) and spices.

Let's take a look at a popular raw food recipe called "Nut Loaf", which is supposed to imitate a meat loaf and which contains, among other things:

- 1 1/3 cups cashews
- 1 1/3 cups sunflower seeds
- 1 1/3 cups almonds
- 1/2 cup oil

This serves two. Let's take a closer look. The fat content of the nuts and oil used in the recipe is as follows:

- Cashews: 1 1/3 cups = 150 grams = 69.5 grams fat
- Sunflower seeds: 1 1/3 cups = 190 grams = 94.2 grams fat
- Almonds: 1 1/3 cups = 200 grams = 104.4 g fat
- Olive oil: 1/2 cup = 125 grams = 125 grams fat.

> TOTAL: 393.1 grams fat
> For each person: 196.55 grams fat!

So, each person consumes almost an entire cup of oil in this recipe! And I have seen people eat more! What would be the consequence of sitting down and drinking a cup of oil?

I highlight an extreme example just to show you how crazy raw-food recipes can get. Raw-foodists should have enough common sense to avoid these recipes. They often don't realize that these combinations are a slippery slope — a steep one — and lead to sheer abuse.

The use of salt, spices, soy sauce, miso, onion, garlic and oil excites the palate and leads to overeating. These are not foods that will give you health and energy. It reminds me of all the products vegetarians have created to replace meat: tofu hot-dogs, veggie burgers and the like. But a real vegetarian doesn't want anything that resembles meat. She is over her meat addiction and is not seeking to replace it with foods that resemble it. Likewise, a raw-foodist doesn't strive to create foods that resemble the popular meals she ate in the past.

The ideal is to limit recipes to a few properly combined ingredients. Dr. Doug Graham has a rule that I like. He calls it the 5-5-5 rule. It means that you should eat meals that take less than 5 minutes to prepare, with a maximum of 5 ingredients, and that cost less than $5. ☺

BOOK BONUS: If you would like know easy raw-food recipes that are really healthy and easy to digest, go to www.rawsecretsbonus.com and click on "Free Book Bonuses". I will give a free subscription to my weekly "Raw Recipe of the Week" Newsletter (a $47 value).

CHAPTER 15

Salt, Spices & Condiments

Pure food can make a poet of you:

> There is nothing that entices us with
> greater appeal, nothing that awakens the
> desire to eat, nothing that arouses every
> organ of digestion and pleases the sense of
> taste more than Nature's richly colored,
> delicately flavored, highly scented,
> luscious and odorous edibles.
>
> He who is accustomed to eating unseasoned,
> unspiced foods knows that condiment users
> are missing many fine, delicate flavors that
> are far more pleasing to the sense of taste
> than any sauce, relish, or spice can ever
> be. Real pleasure in eating comes from
> tasting the natural flavors in foods.
> *Herbert Shelton*

Nature offers us simple foods that taste good without salt, seasonings, condiments, herbs, spices and other flavorings. Unfortunately, most of us have been raised on highly seasoned and salted foods, so we have difficulty returning to a simple, plain diet. We may even view such a diet as ascetic. Raw-foodists may refrain from using ketchup, mustard and the like, but many of them use dried spices, aromatic herbs and even salt. I fell into the same trap for many years, and even included salt and spices in my recipe book *The Sunfood Cuisine*, though I stated that it was possible to make delicious recipes without salt and spices.

I now recommend avoiding these substances. Even though I always knew that these condiments were not the best, it took me a while to realize their true nature. I thought their consequences were negligible. I was wrong!

That being said, it doesn't mean that you have to refuse fanatically to taste something, just because it has some cumin powder in it. It is best to avoid salt and spices without making a religion out of it.

Salt

The body needs sodium, but in small quantities. You get it from the fruits and vegetables you eat. Good tomatoes taste a little salty. Celery, spinach and dark greens are naturally rich in salt. The sodium that natural foods contain is enough to meet your needs. By adding sea salt to your diet, you are almost certain to take in too much sodium and this will lead to several imbalances. Knowing that the body only requires less than 500 mg. of sodium per day (perhaps a little more if you are very active), and that a teaspoon of the best Celtic sea salt contains 1900 mg. of sodium, it is easy to understand how adding sea salt to the diet will create problems fast.

Salt kills life, which is why we preserve foods in salt — it prevents living activity from occurring. It is an antibiotic, which means "anti-life". If you put salt on a fresh cut in your skin, you will be able to feel its effects on yourself. It will burn you.

Salt can accumulate in the body. It causes the body to retain water in order to dilute the salt in the tissues, and to prevent harming the cells. Excess salt is deposited at various places in the body, such as on the walls of the arteries. Blood flow is thereby disrupted, and high blood pressure is the result.

Sea salt is not much better than other types of salt. Sea salt is just rock salt diluted by the ocean. The body has no use for it when it can have access to the natural sodium contained in fruits and vegetables.

Before the Europeans arrived on this continent, native people did not use salt and were in excellent health. Many cultures throughout the world never used salt until the Europeans introduced this poison to them. After they started including salt into their diet, their health progressively deteriorated, although there were several other contributing factors to this deterioration.

Animals don't eat salt, unless they get tempted into licking a salt source somewhere in nature, which rarely happens. Their instinct is better than ours, but not 100% perfect. They can also make mistakes and be fooled by salt. Anyhow, salt licks are rare and most animals never have access to them.

When you stop eating salt, it will take many months for your body to reject it. Some days you may taste salt in your mouth, although you may not have eaten it in weeks. It is another proof that the body is rejecting the salt and not using it. You may urinate more at night for a while, even many months, until the body has rejected all the salt. Complete "desalinization" of the body may take years.

To replace salt, I have come up with a natural seasoning using celery. Simply dehydrate slices of celery (in very large quantities) in a dehydrator or oven (open, at low temperature.) When they are completely dried, turn them into a powder using a coffee grinder. This will make a nice, naturally salty seasoning that you can use to replace salt. You can do the same with other vegetables to add additional flavor to this seasoning. Dried purple cabbage powder is especially good in salads.

Spices

Spices include curry powder, cinnamon, black pepper, cloves, etc. They are made from roots, barks or leaves of different plants. They all taste bitter, hot, or otherwise unpleasant when eaten alone. They are all toxic to some degree. Nutmeg is even a powerful hallucinogen, when eaten in sufficient quantities.

Aromatic Herbs

This category includes all herbs used for cooking: sage, thyme, basil, etc. These plants are too bitter or unpleasant to eat alone. This is because they contain toxic elements. If you go a while without any herbs, spices and salt and then eat them again, you will notice an unusual thirst and maybe even itchiness.

I agree that their scent is fascinating, and their flavor, when mixed with other foods, is pleasant. The occasional use of fresh parsley, basil, dill, or cilantro is okay. But I would avoid oregano, sage, rosemary, thyme and all herbs with a very strong taste.

Raw Garlic, Onions, Leeks

These fresh spices are used raw and cooked all over the world. They contain mustard oil, which, unless oxidized by cooking or long exposure to air, is an irritant that greatly upsets the digestive tract. Some raw-foodists eat a lot of these foods and therefore carry a constant, unpleasant onion odor and breath.

I find that if I eat raw onions and garlic, I will get an unpleasant taste in my mouth hours later. Garlic even comes out from every pore in the body. If you eat garlic one night, you can smell it all over you the next day!

If you like the taste, you can chop some onion or garlic and rinse them with warm water, or dehydrate them to evaporate some of the mustard oil. Also, when chopped in a food processor, onions lose a lot of their mustard oil through oxidation.

If you really like the taste of garlic, you can instead use fresh garlic flowers or garlic greens. They are much milder. To grow garlic greens anywhere, simply plant garlic cloves in some soil (this can be done indoors) and use the greens and flowers of the plant. The same goes for onions.

Hot Peppers

Hot peppers are especially toxic. They contain capsaicin, which is a very poisonous substance. You can easily prove to yourself the toxicity of hot peppers by observing your body's reactions after eating them. The mouth salivates, and the nose often runs with clear mucus or water. These are ways for the body to dilute the poison. The warm feeling that you get is the irritation of the digestive tract and stomach. The body temperature often rises as the body tries to get rid of this strong, toxic substance.

Another argument against hot peppers and spices is that children will refuse them. No one would give a hot pepper to a child. Pregnant and nursing women are advised to avoid them. Apparently, the taste of garlic and onions, and the spiciness of hot peppers can be tasted in milk the day after the mother eats them. I take this to be another proof that the body is rejecting the toxins found in these foods.

At first, when you stop using spices and salt, some foods may taste bland to you. That is because spices and salt greatly dull your senses and your ability to enjoy the natural flavor of natural foods. After a few weeks, you won't even miss spices anymore — and food will taste even better without them. The subtle, intense flavors of natural foods are imperceptible to the dulled palate of the condiment eater.

CHAPTER 16

Food Combining

Simplicity in Eating

In the Garden of Eden, we satisfied our thirst and hunger under the mango tree and ate a few leaves from the plants growing under it. When we felt hunger again, we ate under the fig tree and so on. But going back to that simplicity is very difficult in our complicated world. This is why we need information on how to combine our foods properly, in order to avoid digestive problems.

Quantities of food also matter. Two or three almonds probably combine with anything. When you eat more than two or three, they only combine well with certain foods. And any foods eaten in excess will lead to fermentation and putrefaction, whether they are combined well with other foods or not.

With a simple, mainly raw food diet, you automatically avoid most bad food combinations. In a traditional diet, everything is mixed together in every possible way. Ease of digestion is not the goal, but rather the excitement of the senses within one meal.

Humans originally appreciated the flavors of unadulterated fruits and vegetables. It takes time to learn to eat cooked, spicy, fatty, salted foods, just like it takes time for the smoker to learn to enjoy smoking, and the alcoholic to learn to enjoy whiskey. It will take time to unlearn it and be able to enjoy the natural flavors of fruits and vegetables.

Whenever you combine foods in a dish or during a meal, it must be done in such a way that these combinations digest easily. Bad food combinations create indigestion, fermentation and gas. All these signs, commonly considered normal, are indications of digestive malfunction. The food is fermenting and putrefying in the intestines. Instead of feeding the body, the food poisons it. But you want that food to nourish you, not poison you. So that's why it pays to observe a few simple food-combining rules.

Where Does Food Combining Come From?

Almost a hundred years ago, Dr. Hay, an American physician, started the research on food combining. At the time, no one even suspected that certain foods could cause digestive problems when mixed together. After a series of experiments, he came to the conclusion that protein foods (meat, nuts, cheese, etc.) should be eaten separately from starchy foods (bread, potatoes, etc.), for optimal digestion.

Later came Dr. Shelton, with his methodical and analytic mind. Dr. Shelton first grouped different foods into different categories according to each food's characteristics. He grouped acid fruits together, sub-acid fruits, sweet fruits, starchy foods, and so on.

Dr. Shelton wanted to discover which categories of foods would mix with which others. This was much simpler than trying to test every single food separately. He came up with a series of "rules" or guidelines that have had a considerable impact on many diet theories after him.

Dr. Shelton wrote about food combining in his book *Food Combining Made Easy*. Later the Diamonds, with their book *Fit for Life*, made the food-combining theory available to the masses.

Since then, thousands of food-combining charts have been created, and yet many people are confused about these simple rules. They try to follow them without really understanding them.

Dr. Albert Mosséri of France, who was a student of Shelton's, pointed out that many of Shelton's rules were just based on his experience, not on any particular theory. Mosseri pointed out that it is rather pointless to try to define combining rules for foods that are unhealthy and shouldn't be eaten in the first place.

Mosséri thought that by discussing the combination of foods Shelton himself condemned, he misled a lot of his readers. Shelton never served meat, bread, or grains at his health retreat, but he included them in his food-combining tables.

Mosséri decided to only discuss the combination of foods that are healthy, and not include those that are not part of a hygienic diet. Many hygienists after him (Graham, Klein, etc.) have also created food-combining charts that only included healthy and hygienic fare.

Another criticism made by Mosséri, when he reviewed Shelton's "rules", was that for many of his rules, Shelton gives no explanation at all. In the end, Mosséri found that all these rules were too complicated and discouraged a lot of people.

Shelton also didn't discuss the concept of sequential eating, which is *the order* in which foods are consumed. He didn't believe it was important. But many researchers and nutrition experts who came after Shelton found the concept of sequential eating most useful. It is actually a great complement to food-combining rules.

With sequential eating, you could eat a meal of foods that do not necessarily "combine" without digestive problems, as long you eat the foods in the proper order. We'll talk more about sequential eating in the next chapter.

Food Combining Simplified to Three Simple Rules

I have simplified food combining rules to a few simple rules. Let's take a look at those rules:

1) Do not combine fat with sugar.

This is probably the most important rule to follow. The combination of fat (or protein) with sugar encourages fermentation. But some authors allow combining an acid fruit (such as an orange) with a fat (such as nuts or avocado). The idea is that the acidity in those fruits is appropriate to help digest fats, and the sugar content of these fruits is not as high.

Examples of this bad combination include: dates with nuts, dried fruits with avocado, avocado with sweet fruits, a fruit salad with coconut, etc.

2) Do not combine acid with starch.

Acid with starch is a pretty bad combination. The acidity literally stops the digestion of starches in the mouth, or makes it much more difficult (and sometimes painful.)

Examples of this combination include: mixing tomatoes with (cooked) potatoes, the classic tomato sandwich, and mixing bananas with oranges. Oranges are very acidic and bananas contain starch, even when they are ripe. Bananas combine better with fruits that contain less acidity (sweet apples, mangoes, etc.)

3) Do not combine different types of fatty foods within one meal.

Fatty foods are quite difficult to digest. When many different kinds of fats are present within a meal, digestion is considerably slower.

Examples of this combination include: nuts with avocados, nuts with oil, coconut with avocado, coconut with other types of nuts, etc.

That's it! Those are the basic rules when eating a raw/hygienic diet. Of course, we could come up with more rules, but they would be for combinations that wouldn't be appealing. If you just keep those three rules in mind, you'll overcome most digestive problems people have when attempting to eat a raw food diet.

Clarifications
Here are a few clarifications regarding certain combinations.

Combining Fruits & Green Leafy Vegetables Together

Combining leafy-greens (spinach, lettuce, celery, etc.) with any type of fruit is a good combination. It doesn't break any of our three basic rules. Most people find this combination appealing and it is a fact that it digests well.

A good example of this combination is the *green smoothie* (see appendix).

Combining Various Types of Fruit Together

Simple is better. But if you want to mix different types of fresh fruits together, that's fine. They all combine well together, except for a few that are too concentrated: such as bananas, durian, etc.

Melons

Melons can be combined with other types of fruit without problems. Even Shelton said so in his book, but no one noticed so, they all imposed this rigid rule that "melons should only be eaten alone," which is not true.

What About Dried Fruit?

Dried fruit is not a food that I recommend, so there's no point in discussing its food combining. It doesn't combine well with most acid and sub-acid fruits.

A Few Other Rules

These are combinations for foods that I don't recommend, but the rules are good to know nonetheless:

1) Do not combine cooked starch with sugar.

Cooked starch with sugar is one of the worst combinations possible. No wonder so many people suffer from gas.

Some examples include: bread with jam, cakes and pastries of all kinds, baked beans (with sugar), etc.

2) Do not combine different types of cooked starch together.

Mixing different types of cooked starches together invites digestive confusion.

Some examples include: bread and potatoes, potatoes and pasta, etc.

3) Do not combine proteins with starch.

Some examples include: meat and potatoes, bread and meat, bread and cheese, etc.

These simple rules are the result of scientific observation of human digestive physiology and the experience of thousands of people for two hundred years. If you wish to further explore this interesting topic, there are many excellent books available. I recommend a booklet by Dennis Nelson called *Food Combining Simplified,* as well as *Food Combining Made Easy,* by Dr. Herbert Shelton.

CHAPTER 17

Sequential Eating

Sequential eating is about eating foods in a certain sequence in order to improve digestion. The concept of sequential eating perfectly complements the rules of food combining.

In the last chapter, I broke food combining down to its three most essential rules that apply when eating a raw diet. These rules are:

- Do not mix sugar with fat.
- Do not mix an acid with starch (such as bananas.)
- Do not mix different types of fats together.

In this chapter, I'm going to present the concept of sequential eating, which perfectly complements food-combining rules, and can even "bypass" them in some cases.

Is there a preferred order to eat foods in order to encourage a better digestion? Yes, and you'll see, once you've mastered the concept, your digestion will never be the same. This principle will also help those who have trouble consuming sufficient quantities of fruits and vegetables to be well nourished.

A Little Theory

A food that digests quickly must wait for other foods that digest slowly to leave the stomach. This process can take several hours. During that time, many types of foods (especially fruit and starches) start fermenting, producing gas and even alcohol.

What has been discovered is that when foods are eaten one at a time, the entire meal will digest in different "layers". So, if five different types of food are eaten, one at a time, there could be up to five different types of digestion going on, with enzymes adapting to each particular type of food!

But when the five types of food are eaten altogether, by either mixing everything in the plate or in the mouth, then the stomach is filled with the same mixture, and will take a lot longer to digest, with more difficulties too.

Many physiologists have confirmed the fact that foods digest in different "layers". In one case, a soldier was wounded, with a large opening on his stomach. Several doctors were present and could study the digestion "live", and they observed that his stomach digested foods in different layers.

Watery Foods First

The first concept to understand is that you should always start eating watery foods first and finish with concentrated foods. The watery foods, such as fresh fruit, are digested rapidly, and leave room for the more concentrated foods.

If you eat in any other sequence, which would be to eat concentrated foods first and then watery foods such as fruit, the fruit is more likely to stay in the stomach for too long and ferment.

When you eat a piece of melon on an empty stomach, it digests very rapidly. Within minutes it already exits the stomach. With this understanding, it is then possible to eat something incompatible after this, such as avocado or nuts.

Fruit First

Eat your fruit first, and then have vegetables or more concentrated foods after. Not the other way around. Many people have a big salad or a sandwich and then have a piece of fruit. They then complain that fruit gives them gas. To avoid that, have the fruit first, and then other foods.

Acid Fruit First

Acid fruits include citrus, pineapple, kiwis, tomatoes, etc. Eating those foods at the end of a meal causes indigestion for some people. It's always better to eat them before all other types of fruit.

Some Bad Sequences

- Nuts followed by fruit, or starch
- Starch followed by fruit or starch
- Starch followed by acid foods
- Bananas followed by acid fruits
- Cooked food followed by fruit or nuts
- Dried fruit followed by fresh fruit
- Potatoes followed by tomatoes

Some Good Sequences

- Acid fruits followed by less acid fruits
- Vegetables followed by starch
- Fruit (wait twenty minutes) and then a vegetable soup
- Fruit (wait twenty minutes), and then a salad (with or without fat)
- Melon, followed by other types of fruit

Digestion of Some Foods

This is the time of digestion for some types of food, when they are eaten one at a time, in a small quantity.

<u>Very Fast</u>: Melon, juicy fruit, fruit juice, vegetable juice, vegetable broth, blended salad (without fat)

<u>Fast</u>: Raw vegetables, blended salads (without fat), etc.

<u>Slower</u>: Steamed vegetables, light starches (root vegetables, etc.)

<u>Slow</u>: Grains, bread, avocado, oil, etc.

<u>Very slow</u>: Nuts, protein foods, etc.

To Repeat the Key Principles

- Eat foods ideally one at a time, or one TYPE of food at a time.

- Eat the least dense food first, and the densest last.

- One exception would be to start with nuts or avocado (or another protein food), and then follow with vegetables (but nothing else.) This sequence also digests well, as the vegetables do not have a tendency to ferment.

In conclusion, the ideal remains the natural way: eat one food at a time!

CHAPTER 18

Digestion

Instead of seeking the latest super-food or supplement, or trying various therapies, pay attention to your digestion. When foods putrefy and ferment, they end up poisoning you. Poisons are reabsorbed in the intestines and may be the cause for headaches and many discomforts.

The quality of your digestion depends on many factors, such as your state of mind when eating, what foods are eaten, the degree of hunger, the strength of digestion, food combining, the quantities of food eaten, etc.

Judge Your Digestion

You can judge the quality of your digestion by taking a look at your stools. They should be:

- Quick
- Non-staining (no need for toilet paper)
- Without gas or bad odor

Stools from a healthy human are not as dense, dry, and solid as those of people living on standard fare. They can be loose or dissolve in the toilet bowl — it doesn't matter. They shouldn't have any bad smell or be difficult to pass. A healthy bowel movement literally happens in an instant — a matter of seconds.

Bad-smelling stools, gas, noise in the stomach, pains — which are considered normal — are signs of indigestion. A dried mouth, when living mostly on fruits and vegetables, is also a sign of indigestion.

The quality of your sleep will also depend on digestion. If you eat too much, or eat late at night, your sleep will be disturbed, sometimes by nightmares.

When you wake up in the morning, you should not have any burps, gas, noise in the stomach, or any sign that digestion is still going on in your stomach. If you do, it means digestion went on all night (depriving you of sleep), and is still going on in the morning. In order to correct the situation, fast until you feel true hunger and proceed to eat small amounts of properly combined food.

There are many causes of poor digestion:

- **Eating without hunger** — When the body needs no food and thus gives no signals for it, digestion is ineffective.
- **Poor food combining** — Properly combining your meals will avoid many digestive problems. The mono-eater, who eats one food at a time, enjoys superior digestion.
- **Poor eating conditions** — Eating in a hurry, or in a noisy or polluted atmosphere, hinders digestion. Let us eat when relaxed and in a nice environment. Also, negative emotions — like fear, worry and anxiety — instantly suspend the secretion of digestive juices. Under these conditions, it is imperative that you refrain from eating until you feel relaxed and happy.
- **Overeating** — When overeaten, even the best foods will not digest properly. If you eat too much, you end up digesting little of it.
- **Eating non-specific foods** — Many commonly consumed foods are not meant to be eaten by humans, and thus digest poorly even when properly combined. But when you stick to your natural foods (see Chapter 1) you will be sure to enjoy excellent digestion.

- **Use of salt, spices, and condiments** — These substances are highly toxic. They impair and disturb digestion. Spicy foods are usually rejected, often causing diarrhea.

Assimilation

People worry that the foods they eat do not contain enough minerals. But even the best organic foods bring little to the body if poorly digested. When your digestion works well, you can get all the vitamins and minerals you need from whole natural foods.

CHAPTER 19

Juicing & Blending

Is It Natural?

The position of traditional Natural Hygiene on the subject of juicing is simple: juicing extracts the fiber out of foods, thus making those foods less whole, more refined, and less fit to nourish the body properly. Natural hygienists generally recommend to avoid juicing, and eat whole foods instead.

I tend to agree with that as well. But I also think that some vegetable juices can be very helpful and healthy. I do not attribute to them any special "healing powers", but I see their benefits this way: vegetable juices require virtually no digestion and enable you to get the nutrition from vegetables -- all those important minerals that you need -- in a very absorbable form. This can be a very good help for those with compromised digestion and assimilation.

I still prefer blending to juicing, but I think there can be a place for juicing in a raw-food program. I only recommend vegetable juices — not fruit juices. The sugar in fruit juices is absorbed too quickly when separated from the fiber that comes with it when the fruit is eaten whole.

How to Drink Juices

Green vegetable juices in small quantities can be very beneficial, but avoid drinking large quantities of juices. A few glasses are enough.

The strong green juices (kale, parsley, lettuce, etc.) can be diluted with the milder vegetables: fennel, celery, etc. Some carrot, beet or apple can be used as a flavoring, but not as the main ingredient. The juice can also be diluted with water.

When I make vegetable juices, I often add the pulp back to the juice. What I usually do is drink about 70% of the juice, and then add the rest of the juice back with the pulp. I often eat this mixture with some chopped up tomatoes and avocado. I find this quite delicious and satisfying!

Smoothies and Blended Foods

I believe blended foods to be superior to juices. For this reason, I recommend the consumption of green smoothies (see the appendix or go to www.GreenForLifeProgram.com)

Blended foods are great for getting a concentrated meal that's ready in a minute. You can combine a bunch of fruit and greens with some water and create a tasty "green" smoothie that can be enjoyed anytime as a meal. This is better than juice because you get the fiber, which is an essential nutrient.

The fiber in fruits and vegetables is in the food for many reasons. And "wholesome" means just that: whole. Whole foods are foods as they are found in nature, with nothing added or removed. In our modern world, juicing is a concession that must be used in moderation. Sticking to whole foods is always better.

Carrot Juice

Proponents of carrot juice are numerous. A lot of books have been written hailing carrot juice as a miracle food — the cure for every disease. On the other hand, other authors have accused it of the worst calamities (raising the blood sugar, causing hypoglycemia) because of its high sugar content. Personally, I have nothing against carrots. No one ever showed me sufficient proof that carrots could be dangerous to our health. Carrots are a perfectly respectable root vegetable. But I agree that drinking large quantities of carrot juice is detrimental. But the same goes for any fruit juice: apple, orange, etc. All the benefits attributed to carrot juice could be surpassed by a simple diet of fruits and vegetables.

> ``So, Fred, can I still drink an occasional glass of carrot juice?''

Of course! Why not? But drink a small glass, not a quart. More would be pure excess.

BOOK BONUS: I would like to offer you a series of articles I wrote on the benefits of blended foods and smoothies (versus juicing). To receive this book bonus, go to www.rawsecretsbonus.com and click on "Free Book Bonuses".

CHAPTER 20

The 100% Raw Food Diet

Fanaticism takes most of the credit for dietary self-sabotage. It is through fanaticism that people lose their sense of reality and cannot judge the results of their actions objectively. Obsessed with the idea that a completely raw food diet is the ultimate diet, raw-foodists sometimes forget the bigger picture.

Although correct 100% raw eating is great, the way some raw-foodists eat is not necessarily healthy, as we have seen. Simply because a meal is raw doesn't mean it's going to be healthy. A 100% raw food diet only works when done correctly.

I have met many people who were raw-foodists for two or three years and then went back to eating the SAD (Standard American Diet) because of constant cravings and dissatisfaction. Wouldn't it have been better to figure out something more sustainable, instead of going back to meat and bread?

Raw and Unheated: Not the Same

There is big difference between what is raw and what is merely unheated. According to the dictionary, raw, in addition to meaning "uncooked" means, "not processed, purified or refined". Raw food is food in its natural state — whole fruits, vegetables, nuts and seeds. This is my definition of "raw". Oils, dried fruit, dehydrated crackers, etc., could be unheated, but are they truly "raw?"

I don't consider the following foods to be truly raw, that is, completely unadulterated, even though some of them are technically unheated: most store-bought nuts and seeds, dried foods, oils or coconut butter, most nut butters, dried spices, herbs and frozen fruit.

How many raw-foodists eat foods from the list above? Most of them, I would say. So why make a big fuss about 100% raw when lots of the foods they hail as raw are not? Instead of constantly worrying about raw, think in terms of health. Ask yourself, "Is this really healthy for me?" "Do I feel great after eating it?" "Is it a specific food for humans?" "Is this a fruit?" "Is this a vegetable?" "Is this easily digestible?"

So, really, when we talk about a 100% raw food diet, we mean mostly raw. We mean a diet that avoids heating foods, but unless one only eats only fresh raw fruits, vegetables, nuts and seeds — without making any exceptions, this diet is not truly 100% raw.

I personally have gone long periods of time on either a 100% unheated diet or 100% raw food diet. I do not claim to eat 100% raw all the time, and I do not pretend that I'll even "become" 100% raw one day. I eat this way for health and energy, and make as few compromises as I possibly can, but I am not perfect either. I tend to go long periods of time (during the summer), on raw foods only. But there are also times where I'll eat some cooked foods, such as steamed vegetables.

I have found that I enjoy more energy eating raw foods, so I stick to raw foods as much as possible. But from having been a little extreme about the raw food diet in the past, I am now more relaxed about it.

Raw Is Not the Only Criterion

We must have common sense and be aware that not everything raw is better than anything cooked. I consider steamed vegetables to be easier on the body than large quantities of nuts and seeds.

I also consider the "junk food" category (pizza, chips, fried foods, coffee, ice cream and pastries) to be worse than meat. So, a piece of chicken with a salad is not as bad as a slice of pizza with a salad.

Our *ideal* foods are fresh fruits and vegetables — fresh produce (including fresh nuts and seeds.) These are our true natural foods. Everything else is a concession to the artificial world we live in.

A Rational Approach

It is impossible to be 100% right or 100% strict. Beware of militant proposals. I knew people who, after years of eating a 100% raw food diet, were dreaming of eating huge chocolate cakes. But if someone has dreams like that, it means he is not satisfied with what he eats. I hope that, by reading this book, you get good ideas on how to balance your diet and make it more satisfying and sustainable.

Many raw-foodists either cheat or make mistakes. What types of mistakes can be made on a 100% raw food diet? They are numerous and have been reviewed in this book. Here is a summary:

Common Mistakes Made by Raw-Foodists

- Use of salt, condiments, spices
- Eating too many avocados, or even eating avocados every day
- Eating too many nuts or nut butter
- Constantly worrying and thinking about food
- Drinking large quantities of juices, especially fruit juices
- Eating honey, maple syrup, or other concentrated sweets
- Using raw cacao —the fact that it's raw doesn't make it less toxic
- Eating a raw food diet except for drinking coffee or tea
- Eating lots of sprouted beans and grains
- Sleeping too little, or at irregular hours
- Paying no attention to digestion, dismissing hygienic food combining and eating complex mixtures
- Overeating greens by dulling the taste with gourmet salads

- Eating raw, but not taking care of your dental health
- Eating raw, but not paying attention to hunger
- Eating raw, but not exercising
- Eating raw, but spending too much time in the sun
- Overeating acid fruit
- Eating dried fruit
- Eating dates on a regular basis
- Using oils on a regular basis

Some 100% raw-foodists don't cheat and don't make these mistakes. They feel balanced and healthy. Superb! Keep on. I would not recommend any changes to these people. I am proposing a raw food diet — all raw, or close to it, done correctly; but I think it's time to get rid of these fantasies that a 100% raw food diet is the solution to everything; that it can work easily in all cases and situations. The experience of many raw-foodists throughout the world proves that a raw food diet is very beneficial — but it's not the only factor in health, or the most important, and it cannot be done recklessly.

It's not a sin to eat a few steamed vegetables occasionally, if you feel that you can't stick to a 100% raw food diet at this point or if you just want to get some benefits from eating raw, without going all the way. Not all cooked foods are equal. Steamed vegetables are easy on the body and will not wear you down like other cooked foods (bread, pasta, meat, etc.)

You can easily limit yourself to fruits and vegetables without going into grains, bread and meat. Steamed vegetables certainly better than high-fat, raw recipes, which, in my opinion, are "gateway foods" to worse things.

Is 100% Raw Easier?

Eating 100% raw, or close to it, is actually easier than eating 70% raw. When you are ready and start to eat all raw, your desire to eat cooked food goes away after a few weeks. That is, of course, if you pay attention to all the factors I have reviewed in this book.

Although eating an all-raw diet is within the reach of almost everyone who wants it, some people may not have the health, or the mental and physical constitution, to do it right now. They will need a well-planned transition. A competent Hygienic practitioner would never recommend an all-raw diet to everyone immediately, in every single case. Diet has to be adapted to people's needs, rather than blindly conforming to an ideal.

CHAPTER 21

The Psychology of Dietary Change

When you try to follow a healthy diet, it's perfectly normal at first to have desires or cravings for unhealthy foods and to feel tempted by those foods. Sometimes, for one reason or another, you may decide to say "What the hell!" and indulge.

First, it should be said that what matters most is what you do on a daily basis and not what you do rarely or occasionally. So, small dietary deviations once in a while are not as harmful as they would be if they were habitual. The other side of the coin is that *these small but repeated cheats can sabotage all the benefits you are expecting to receive from your diet.*

When you eat a diet composed mostly of fruits and vegetables without spices or salt, and when you eat those foods with genuine hunger, you eventually purify your body and become more sensitive to any poor food choice. The body reacts to any unhealthy food, much like a child's body.

The worst thing is the surprise of finding out that the old foods you used to love -- those that seem so innocent still -- can have such a dramatic effect on you. You'd like to be able to eat them occasionally and be fine... oh, you'd like so much to be able to!

Let me use my own experience as an example.

In most people's minds, a cooked vegan meal is a rather healthy meal. Most folks would eat that and feel fine. That might even be the healthiest thing they ate all week! But for someone whose system has been cleansed out by a pure diet of fruits and vegetables, things aren't the same.

If I ate such a meal, let's say, composed of split pea soup, a vegan pizza and soy ice cream, it would definitely affect me in the most negative way. I might have a hard time falling asleep and my sleep could be disturbed by weird dreams. I'd become dehydrated from all the salt in those "healthy" vegan foods. But the worst thing is that I'd have such a hard time getting back on track again. For a week I might feel kind of ill, but not really fall ill— just a sort of slight sore throat and aching in the muscles. A slight depression could even set in and I'd have the hardest time getting to feel like myself again. What a setback for just a little dietary indiscretion!

I know from experience what happens when I decide to eat something I normally don't eat, having been there more than a few times. But I also know that this experience is common to all those that have experienced living on a natural diet of fruits and vegetables.

Studying the Law of Vital Adaptation will help you understand why this happens.

Here is the law, as stated by Herbert Shelton: *"The response of the vital organism to external stimuli is an instinctive one, based upon a self-preservative instinct which adapts itself to whatever influence it cannot destroy or control."*

What it means is that over time, the body can become accustomed to all sorts of harmful substances. It will adapt itself to them in order to protect itself. This is done at the expense of many vital processes. Shelton again said:

"There was the ancient king who, in order to protect himself against poisoning by his foes, accustomed his body to various poisons by a

gradual increase in the amount taken, until, when a time finally arrived when he desired to take his own life, by poisoning, he failed in the attempt. *The first effort of the living organism, in relation to adverse and inimical influences, is to overcome and destroy them. Failing in this, it attempts to accommodate itself to such conditions and influences. For what it cannot overcome, it must learn to endure or perish."*

When we start a pure diet of fruits and vegetables, the process described by Shelton is done in reverse. *The body rejects accumulated toxins and reverts to a more pure state that has little tolerance for poisons.* That is why you can now react so strongly to the foods you used to eat without a second thought.

It's a Learning Process

It's a rather interesting experience to see how bad certain foods can make you feel once you've eaten a simple diet of mostly fruits and vegetables for a while. I've noticed how certain foods make you drowsy, others just stimulate you and later make you feel depressed, others make you feel irritated, and others make you feel almost drugged.

A friend of mine isn't a habitual coffee drinker. Recently, he had four coffees in one evening. Although he felt great initially, because of stimulation, the following day he fell into a sort of depression that lasted a good two days!

This backsliding is probably necessary to understand where you want to go. But what really hurts in the long term are the small cheats that end up occurring on a rather regular basis. Let me explain. If you go out one night and have a pizza after having been on a clean diet for a while, you will feel it. I guarantee that you will not feel encouraged to repeat the experience the next day. But if instead you have a muffin here and there, drink some tea once in a while, add some soy sauce to your salads, etc., you might not feel horrible, but all of those little things begin to add up and one day you wonder why you don't feel so good anymore, without realizing what has actually happened.

Taking It Easy

Life should be fun, and eating healthy shouldn't be a big struggle. At some point, you have to accept the path that you have chosen and be happy with it. What's the point of eating healthy if you feel deprived and you're constantly going back and forth and trying to find your balance again each time?

Trying to eat raw using force of willpower alone will ultimately fail. On one side you are trying to make yourself eat in a way that you think is good for you, but on the other side you are fighting it, because on that level you do not want to do it. This inner struggle, in spite of the greatest willpower in the world, is going to make you fail.

The key is to come to accept on a deeper level the diet choice you have made, rather than understand it on a purely intellectual level. I always tell people that they shouldn't strive to eat a particular diet, such as a raw food diet, simply because they think it's the best for their bodies. Instead, they should write down their reasons they are doing it. The reasons can include: having more energy, improved complexion, waking up feeling energetic, feeling more connected to nature, feeling more peaceful inside, radiating health, living healthfully, etc.

Everything in Balance

A discrepancy between what we eat and who we are in the world generates a kind of tension, which is resolved either when the diet moves back in line with the person's incarnate role, or when the person's entire life changes to come in harmony with the new diet. Force, that is, willpower, can hold diet and being apart, but not forever. The tension will build, in the form of intense cravings, aversions, and, eventually, physical illness.

> Charles Eisenstein, The Yoga of
> Eating

One thing that took me a long time to understand is that your diet must harmonize with your other behaviors; otherwise it is doomed to fail. There's a saying that goes, "You cannot change one thing without changing everything." Let me explain.

A diet of animal foods and alcohol is compatible with a number of lifestyles, but incompatible with some others. The same holds for a vegan diet, or a raw-food diet.

A raw plant-based diet, such as the one described in *The Raw Secrets*, is a radical change. It will call for more radical changes in every area of your life. If you are not ready for it and were just looking for a quick fix, you will have to face some major hurdles along the way, because your diet choice won't harmonize with your other manners of being.

A fruit-based diet is a high-energy diet. It isn't compatible with a sedentary lifestyle. It isn't compatible with certain low-energy activities, friendships, and even jobs.

So one way to make the diet work, indirectly, is to focus on other areas of your life. Instead of focusing on the diet, you can focus on becoming more active, or inviting new, more positive friendships. By harmonizing those areas of life, it will become easier to make the diet work almost effortlessly.

CHAPTER 22

Binges and Cravings

The scene is familiar. You have been "pure" for many weeks. You feel great. You feel confident. But one day, you are tempted to try a piece of something forbidden. Everything goes well, of course, because you only ate a little bit — of cheese, chocolate or bread. But the next day, the thought is there, troubling and unwavering — that chocolate requires another sampling. This time, you eat a little more. You feel a little drunk with the excitement of doing something forbidden, like the teenager smoking in the garage. However, the third day, in spite of your best efforts, you fall and hard. An abominable binge of bread, chocolate, cheese and chips follows. And the worst part of it? You get little pleasure from it, but you can't seem to stop yourself. After that, it takes you weeks to get back on track — feeling morose, sick and angry with yourself.

Binging Common Among Raw-Foodists: An Open Secret

Binging is quite common among raw-foodists. When it's not with cooked food, it's with dried fruits, nuts, and combo-abombos. There are many reasons for this -- some psychological, some physical. Part of it is out of a frustration that arises from eating a diet you are unaccustomed to. Part of it is out of a real, physiological imbalance. Let's see what Mosséri has to say about it:

> It is deplorable that most hygienists only
> observe and expose the lamentable situation

[of binging] in their followers, without trying to find the reasons or analyze the causes. "I was a small eater," a poet told me. "But after switching to the hygienic diet, I became a bulimic overeater!" This situation is unfortunately very common and even almost general among our followers. Let us examine the matter and find a reasonable remedy for it.

There is the overeating that affects those with psychological problems and the overeating that occurs after dietetic mistakes. Armed with the best intentions, we often fall in the trap of overeating, without wanting it and without being able to avoid it. We often find this situation nowadays among Sheltonians and instinctos.

The followers of the latter method take a plant laxative every day — cassia. The foods eaten are rejected the next day in abundant stools and do not benefit the body. This is why their cells are constantly hungry and the person becomes bulimic. For those that are not aware of it, instinctotherapy is the new fad which consists of following our instinct when choosing foods, smelling them and tasting them, according to our desire of the moment, whether we are hungry or not. But before selecting foods with the sense of smell, often distorted, is it not better to wait to be hungry? It seems more important to me. But the followers of this vogue eat without being hungry, according to their caprice. In effect, those who follow this method justify their eating nuts and seeds, meat and fish, on the basis of their sense of smell. But there are also Sheltonian hygienists who eat too many nuts and seeds. These concentrated protein foods are impossible to digest when consumed in excess, and are eliminated in putrescent stools the next day. We don't benefit from any of what we eat, which is why we are always hungry and start binging. Shelton used to say that an excess of fruit gives a small diarrhea in his followers. This is true when nuts and seeds are eaten, in the quantities he recommended, that is, a large handful (four to five ounces). But if we never eat nuts, or eat them in small amounts, we never get diarrhea when we eat too much fruit. The reason is that nuts are so hard to digest that they end up weakening digestion itself and intoxicating the blood. Consequently, we must not make the mistake of saying that diarrhea is caused by an excess of fruits, when it is the nuts and seeds.

I have pointed out the main cause of overeating in Hygienists and instinctos: the over-consumption of nuts and seeds in both and the eating of unnatural foods without hunger, followed by a daily laxative in the latter. We can see that the situation of the instincto is the worse of the two. Their overeating reaches heights never known in human history.

> *À la Recherche d'une Santé Parfaite.*

Mosséri points to the over-consumption of nuts and seeds as being the main reason why hygienists and instinctos become bulimic and indulge in binges. Obviously, it applies to raw-foodists as well. I have found this to be true. Eating a large amount of nuts or other types of fats doesn't really feed you. Rather, it fosters malnutrition. The next day you are hungry, craving anything.

Binges and Cravings .... **THE RAW** SECRETS

Another food that fosters cravings is dried fruit and dates. The over consumption of these foods is quite common among raw-foodists. The concentrated sugar they contain is very hard to digest — even when dried fruit is soaked in advance. They ferment, cause gases, and foster deep cravings. I personally recommend avoiding those foods. I try to eat only dates when they are really juicy and in season, that is only in September/October.

There are many more causes to this overeating, not just the abuse of nuts and seeds. Eating without hunger is a common cause. When you eat without hunger, little is digested, and you are hungry because the body was not well fed. It's a vicious cycle that must be broken.

The Right Attitude

You must cultivate the right, balanced attitude towards food. Moderation is possible in everything — even when going off-track. There are levels of dietary deviations, the small ones and the big ones. Most raw-foodists and natural hygienists seem to fall for the big ones. When they stray off their diet, you'd better watch out. They are like monsters unleashed! In their minds, a calming monologue may be going on to justify their excesses: "You can fast tomorrow." "You already went too far, you might as well enjoy it." "If I'm going to crash, I may as well burn." "It's not so bad, people eat like that every day," and so on.

Most of us have gone through these binges. Perhaps they are necessary to help us understand the damage caused by our previous diet. But the main problem caused by these indulgences is that they upset our instinct, our balance (which is restored slowly) even if you make only regular "tiny exceptions". After that, you stop getting pleasure from unseasoned, natural foods and start looking forward to spices and stimulants to excite your confused palate.

Cravings

Cravings are of another nature. Cravings may lead to binges, but binges do not necessarily follow cravings. Binges may follow a simple taste of food, as described at the beginning of this chapter.

Cravings are a conscious physical or psychological desire for a particular food or substance. They are often a withdrawal symptom and do not reflect physiological need. For example, an ex-smoker may feel a craving for cigarettes, which should not be mistaken for a real need by the body. A coffee drinker, after giving up coffee, will crave coffee for a while until the body has detoxified all the poisons from coffee. Similarly, when giving up salt, bread, spices, pasta, meat, etc., the body may crave these substances for a period, during which temptation must be resisted, with great will, and at all costs.

Psychological cravings are different — they may appear in an ex-coffee drinker, for example, after years of abstinence, simply by entering a coffee shop and smelling coffee. At these times, old images and associations with coffee are triggered in the mind. Basically, one has to snap out of the trance, recognize that the environment is triggering this desire, and either dismiss it in the midst of the environment, or - if it is too strong - leave.

Psychological cravings can occur in cycles. You can be free from them for a while, and then they can hit you with an attack!

However, after a few months on a healthy diet, it is not normal to constantly feel these cravings. In these cases, I attribute craving to poor nutrition and a deranged assimilation, which is usually caused in raw-foodists by any of the following: an excess of fat, dried or sweet fruit, salt intake, eating without hunger, the use of spices, etc.

Not Eating Enough

Many people have never become completely balanced on a strict raw-food diet. After a few years, they still crave cooked food and sometimes fall into avocado, dried fruit, or cashew binges.

A frequent reason for this is that those people do not consume enough calories (energy) from fruit.

Eventually, this deficit will manifest itself in the form of intense cravings. It is imperative to learn to consume enough fruit at a meal, so you are not hungry again for another four to five hours. Otherwise, any mental effort to avoid frustration and hunger will lead to another binge. (It's also important to understand that fruit has a much higher water content compared to cooked starches such as bread and pasta. The quantities of fruit that are consumed on this diet will seem huge at first.)

CHAPTER 23

When to Eat

The following article is translated from Albert Mosséri's book, *À la Recherche d'une Santé Parfaite* (The Quest for Perfect Health).

"Those who adopt the hygienic diet start, with the strongest of wills, to modify their eating habits. They were used to eating small quantities of concentrated foods that fill us up, as we say. Being difficult to digest, they stick to the stomach for hours. These foods are bread, rice, and grains (croissants, rice, granola, cakes, pasta, etc.) The new hygienic eater replaces them with similar quantities of foods that digest easily and leave the stomach in little time, like fruits and vegetables (raw or cooked). So one or two hours after such a meal, these people experience an empty stomach. They take this for 'hunger,' especially if they are not used to eating large quantities of these new foods."

"Confused by this "hunger," which occurs outside of the fixed meal schedule, and getting poor advice from those who tell them not to eat between meals, they feel guilty about wanting to eat and are tormented by this persistent hunger. Then they jump on all the forbidden foods and eat them in large quantities.

"A lady recently told me that she has a small stomach and that she cannot eat a lot of fruit or raw vegetables at one sitting. One hour after such a meal, she is hungry. It is normal. Should she wait many hours to eat at 'meal time?' No. She must eat again, even if the number of meals reaches seven a day, *as long as she waits for hunger each time.*

"In all my previous writings, and for more than thirty years, I have followed the pioneer hygienists, especially Shelton, who recommended two meals a day. However, I now realize that this has been a mistake. In fact, it's the hard-to-detect mistake so many eccentric natural hygienists make.

Fixed Meal Times

> Don't eat just because it's mealtime. If you wait for hunger and are hungry at 10 a.m., for example, but would like to eat at noon with someone, well, it won't hurt you to wait for another two hours. It's not so bad to be hungry. We shouldn't avoid hunger like we would avoid a tiger. Hunger doesn't need to be satisfied at the precise minute. Most people literally fear to be hungry, as if it were a sign of poverty or a sin, or death would fall on them if they did not eat at the first signs of hunger. No one will think that you live in misery, in poverty and in lack if you skip a meal, or if you don't eat every hour.
> *Dr. Virginia Vetrano*

"She's right. So many people are afraid of hunger, as if it were a sign of imperative and urgent need.

"On the other hand, I'm noticing that Dr. Vetrano still talks, like Shelton, about skipping a meal. But I reject the idea of fixed meal times. I repeat that, in my opinion, it's better to wait for hunger than to skip a meal. The first injunction is negative and frustrating, whereas the second is positive and hopeful."

"Two remarks have to be made. Firstly, if we are occupied when we feel the first signs of hunger, we don't even notice it. Secondly, concerning certain very emaciated persons in a state of undernourishment, the first sensations of hunger are accompanied by an extreme weakness — a sensation of fainting. These people must eat something immediately. For this, they must always carry some food with them, in case they leave their house."

Can We Eat at Night?

Hunger is rarely felt at night, with some exceptions, such as during a long fast or in cases of undernourishment. It follows that we should never eat late at night. However, a fast can be broken at anytime, including during the night, with a piece of fruit. Those in a state of undernourishment can also eat a piece of non-acid fruit at night.

Digestion in the stomach cannot continue properly at night. At night, all the muscles of the body loosen up, including the stomach. The consequence is, the stomach cannot energetically mix foods taken during the night. It is the same for the various glands that must secrete the digestive juice. At night, they rest.

"There is a basic rhythm — day and night — that must be respected in your lifestyle. It is the same for plants. If we water them at the wrong moment, or don't water them when they need it the most, they wither away.

"For human beings, night is meant for catabolism and elimination, whereas the day is for anabolism and digestion. These functions should not be inverted by transforming day into night and night into day.

"Hunger can announce itself early in the morning or many hours after waking up. We must wait for it before eating."

CHAPTER 24

Foods of Our Biological Design

Fruit

Like orangutans, bonobos and chimpanzees, humans are frugivores. A frugivore is a fruit eater. Being a frugivore doesn't mean eating only fruit. All these noble animals include green vegetables, as well as nuts and seeds, in their fruit-based diets.

Some say that fruit-based diets are dangerous because of the high amount of sugar they contain. They recommend a calorie-rich diet based on fatty, protein-rich or starchy foods. Fruit is also a source of calories (energy) in the form of simple sugar, which some people confuse with harmful, refined sugar. Let's look at the different possible sources of energy and decide what types of food should form the basis of our diet.

A high-fat diet is a disaster. Excess fat (raw or cooked) reduces oxygen in the blood and leads to several health problems. It causes blood sugar imbalances by decreasing the effectiveness of insulin in carrying sugar to the cells, leading to high blood sugar. Eating too much fat leaves us tired all the time, because fat is difficult to digest. The problems related to the high-fat diet are numerous and well documented.

A high-protein diet is even more dangerous, because excess proteins commonly putrefy during digestion. It poisons the body and lays the foundation for cancer. For these reasons, almost no modern health specialist recommends fat-based or protein-based diets. Sometimes protein-based diets (e.g., the Atkin's diet) are recommended for weight loss. But almost no one considers this type of diet healthy.

Experts generally recommend high-carbohydrate diets. Starch-based carbohydrates include potato, bread, pasta, etc. The advantage to these foods is that they provide energy in the form of complex sugar while being low in fat. The problem is that grains tend to predominate in these diets. As we have learned, grains are not the best foods for human beings. A grain-based diet will acidify the system, as these foods contain very few alkaline minerals. A high-starch diet can work if it consists of cooked root vegetables such as potatoes, yams and manioc, which are alkaline-forming.

When we eat complex carbohydrates (starch), the body must convert the starch into simple sugar. Ultimately, we get energy from simple sugars. Fruit is rich in a special type of simple sugar, which is metabolized easily. Fruit is also alkaline-forming and richer in nutrients than starchy foods. In addition, fruit can be eaten raw. All the vitamins, minerals, and enzymes stay intact and are not destroyed by cooking.

We therefore can draw the conclusion that fruit should dominate the diet. Fruits are rich in vitamins, but sometimes low in certain minerals, such as calcium and sodium, which are abundant in vegetables. This is one reason that vegetables, especially the green leafy ones, are essential.

The fruit we get in stores is also quite different from fruit found in the wild. Store-bought fruit has been hybridized to appeal to the tastes of our ancestors and the increasingly perverse tastes of the modern masses. These fruits contain more sugar, less fiber and fewer minerals and vitamins. Often it has been picked unripe. Even so, it is still better than the rest of the food found in supermarkets.

Some people think we should avoid hybridized fruits, such as pineapple, bananas, seedless grapes and Fuji apples. However, they don't acknowledge that the other commercial fruits, such as mangoes (the best-selling fruit in the world), cherimoyas, and papayas are also hybridized. Not only those, but all of the vegetables and everything else in the store, for that matter is hybridized. So should we eat nothing? I think it is legitimate to want to get natural, organic produce. But we must not make a religion out of it. People are not sick because they eat seedless watermelon. They don't get cancer because they eat Fuji apples. They don't get heart disease because they eat seedless grapes every morning. How about some common sense?

Green Vegetables

All frugivorous creatures eat green leaves and other vegetables. Green leaves are rich in minerals, while fruits are rich in vitamins. Green leafy vegetables include cabbage, lettuce, kale, parsley and spinach, among thousands of others.

To get all of the minerals that you need, you should eat approximately one or two pounds of green leafy vegetables every day.

There are a few challenges with eating a sufficient quantity of green vegetables. First of all, we often do not chew them long enough, and second of all, we don't have time to eat large salads!

The best way to solve this problem is to learn to make green smoothies and blended salads. A green smoothie is simply a fruit smoothie with some green vegetables (spinach, celery, etc.) thrown in there. The result is a surprisingly tasty and nutritious smoothie that is probably the best raw food meal ever.

BOOK BONUS: I would like to offer you a series of articles I wrote on the benefits of blended greens and green smoothies. To receive this book bonus, go to www.rawsecretsbonus.com and click on "Free Book Bonuses".

Fruit-Vegetables

A lot of fruits are not very sweet. Some of these are cucumbers, tomatoes, squash, zucchini and bell pepper. Although those are fruits botanically, we class them as vegetables for their nutritional value and culinary use. They are all excellent foods to eat at any time of the day. Some people react to tomatoes and should consume them in moderation.

Root Vegetables

Root vegetables include carrot, parsnip, Jerusalem artichoke, potato, sweet potato, yam, manioc and celeriac. They are all excellent foods. Some of them can be eaten raw, while others, the more starchy ones, will be more digestible if lightly steamed. Starchy root vegetables cannot be compared to starchy grains. They have none of the problems of starchy grains.

Several indigenous tribes live mainly on cooked root vegetables and are in excellent health — no dental problems, no diabetes, etc. But these diseases appear in these people as soon as bread and other "civilized" foods are introduced. Cooked starchy roots are superior to grains and may comprise 10-25% of the diet during transition. When everything is eaten raw, the less starchy roots can be used. Celeriac is especially good raw.

Nuts and Seeds

In Chapter 4, I warned against eating nuts and seeds in excess. This is a mistake many raw-foodists make. This being said, it doesn't mean that nuts and seeds shouldn't be eaten. They are a part of our natural diet. Nuts found in the wild are delicious seasonal foods; cultivated nuts are not so far from their wild ancestors.

I have noticed that some people seem to fare better with nuts and seeds, while some exclude them entirely without problems. Others have to avoid them for a long period of time, until their digestion improves. At some point, they can start eating them in very small quantities.

In order to be digested properly, nuts have to be chewed very, very well. Nut butters can be useful because they are emulsified and easy to digest, as long as they are made from raw nuts in a process that doesn't generate heat. As far as I know, very few companies market "really raw" nut butters. One source that I highly recommend is Living Tree Community (www.livingtreecommunity.com). Nuts and seeds can also be blended with other foods, such as tomatoes, to make a dressing.

Wild Plants

Edible wild plants grow everywhere. Most of them are quite nutritious, containing an abundance of vitamins and minerals. They have not been hybridized, are freely available, and are strong, sturdy plants. For this reason, a lot has been written on the benefits of eating wild plants.

Wild plants contain more minerals and vitamins than cultivated vegetables. Because of this potency, it is not possible to eat a lot of them. Small, regular quantities of edible wild plants are very beneficial. Eating them in excess is not.

Edible wild plants may be eaten, as long as they taste good to you. If you find them too bitter, you shouldn't force yourself to eat them. Think of the child or animal that has not been quite so corrupted by our twisted ways of thinking. They will never force themselves to eat something that tastes bad, if they could.

I find that some wild plants taste too bitter. Other wild plants such as purslane, young dandelion leaves, milk thistle, sorrel, and lambs quarter, have a pleasant taste.

It should also be mentioned that the same species of plant can taste very different depending on the age of the plant, the condition of the soil, the climate, humidity, etc. Dandelion greens can range from being quite inedible to being positively sweet.

I think we can also benefit from including wild plants in our diet. But never force yourself to overeat them just because you think they are good for you.

Dried Fruits

I don't consider dried fruits to be raw foods, and I don't recommend their consumption, except in exceptional circumstances, when fresh fruit is not available. Exceptional circumstances would be for example, a trip to Antarctica, a long hike in the forest, or crossing the Sahara desert. Then you could bring some dried fruit along and eat it.

Raw-foodists tend to eat too much dried fruit; that, along with the abuse of fat and the other mistakes I have pointed out in this book, is where most of their problems lie. Dried fruits are addictive and most people have a tendency to overeat them. This has bad consequences: gas, indigestion, frequent urination, digestive discomforts, cravings, and disturbed sleep. Dried fruits also stick to the teeth and encourage tooth decay. Many people have ruined their teeth with the consumption of raisins, dates, dried figs, etc. In my case, it was certainly one of the major causes of the cavities I got while on the raw food diet.

If you are craving dried fruit, it is simply due to the fact that you are not eating enough fresh fruit to meet your caloric needs. When you start eating more fresh fruit, all of your cravings for dried fruit will go away. In fact, if you are craving *anything* sweet (other than fresh fruit), you are simply not eating enough fruit.

Since we talked about dried fruit, I must also mention dates. The date is a dried fruit, but it has not been dried artificially. It has dried naturally on the plant. For that reason, I still classify it as a dried fruit.

Dates are renowned as the junk food of the raw-foodist. Most people tend to overeat them. Overeating dates means eating more than five to ten dates at once. Because dates are extremely concentrated in sugar, they will cause the same problems as eating too much dried fruit. For that reason, I do not recommend dates on a regular basis.

I buy dates only a few times a year, at the height of the season, when I can find a certain type of juicy date at the markets. Those dates are only available a few weeks a year, max. Other than then, I do not buy them so I won't get tempted. ☺

Frozen Fruit

Frozen fruits are not completely "raw", but the freezing process preserves most nutrients. The main problem with frozen "raw" foods is that they are eaten cold, which is the equivalent of putting an ice pack inside the stomach. It is almost certain to cause indigestion, and the regular consumption of cold, frozen fruits can negatively affect the state of the bacterial flora and cause a vitamin B12 deficiency.

Frozen fruit can be quite useful when you live in the North like me. Throughout the winter, I use frozen berries (especially wild blueberries). They're really good in smoothies and allow a little extra variety.

However, I recommend thawing frozen fruits before using them, or at least not make a meal out of them. For example, you could make a banana smoothie with fresh bananas and some frozen berries. That way, the entire meal is not frozen. But it's still best to wait an hour or two and let the frozen fruits thaw.

Milk

That humans need to drink the milk of another animal, after being weaned from their own mothers, is an idea so bizarre that it makes me smile. This idea is not based on anything scientific. Rather, it is the spawn of a well-planned, well-executed, decades-long propaganda campaign by the dairy industry. Cow's milk naturally carries powerful growth hormones that are deeply disturbing to the human body. Commercial milk is also loaded with antibiotics, bacteria, pesticides, and cholesterol. It takes ten pounds of milk to make one pound of cheese, so this cornucopia of toxic elements is even more concentrated in cheese than in plain milk.

Contrary to the propaganda, drinking milk will not prevent osteoporosis. The 1995 Harvard Nurses' Health Study, conducted on more than 75,000 women, showed that those getting much of their calcium from milk experience more fractures compared to those drinking little or no milk. Another study done in 1994 in Sydney, Australia, showed much the same thing — higher consumption of dairy products was associated with increased fracture risk. Those who consumed the most dairy products doubled their risk of hip fracture, compared to those who ate fewer dairy products. Other studies have shown that high protein consumption is associated with an increased incidence of osteoporosis.

Animal milk is for that animal's young, and not for humans. All species stop drinking milk after a certain age, and we are no exception. But the milk industry tries to convince us that cow's milk is "nature's perfect food", and that we must never be weaned! It is indeed a perfect food — for baby cows!

Nonetheless, raw goat's or cow's milk can be useful in the case of women who cannot nurse long enough, for whatever reason, or if the milk produced by the mother isn't adequate. Vegan mothers who give soy milk to their children are mistaken. Soymilk cannot replace real milk for growing children, because it is lacking in too many essential nutrients.

Adults cannot digest milk well because the enzymes that digest milk stop being produced after the age of seven or eight. Drinking milk past that age can lead to health problems.

Yogurt

When it is fermented and clabbered (like yogurt or kefir), milk is much more digestible. Natural hygienists have often used natural yogurt when patients could not digest nuts well. So yogurt is easier to digest, however there are many more problems with dairy products than those that could be caused by not being able to digest milk. For more information, go to www.notmilk.com

Honey

Honey is a perfect food for the bees, but not a perfect food for humans. Certainly, commercial honey is very detrimental and akin to white sugar in so many ways.

Honey from pristine a environment is of course better, but it doesn't qualify as a "natural food for humans." When you eat the quantities of fruit I recommend in this book, you won't ever be craving honey or any concentrated sweets.

In certain circumstances I could consider the use of honey, but not as a regular part of the diet. These circumstances might be a long trip to a remote location where carrying a lot of fruits and vegetables would be difficult, or being offered by Balinese locals the tastiest, molasses-tasting wild honey from the jungle (which actually happened to me!), a treat only a very strict vegan could refuse...

Eggs

Eggs have to be stolen from birds, so they are probably not natural foods for humans, although some serious researchers, like Dr. Gian-Cursio, see a lot of benefits in eating the yolks.

Personally, a raw egg yolk doesn't draw me like piece of avocado. On some occasions, I might have egg yolks if they come from animals who have been fed their natural foods only (seeds, vegetables, etc.), and not the abominations that that are fed to even "organic" chicken.

However, I have not done that for many years. I personally prefer the vegan diet.

In the past, I've had the occasion of tasting duck egg yolks from animals fed only natural seeds and vegetables, and I must say the taste was very pleasant.

So, on the topic of egg yolks, I don't see them as something that could be consumed regularly, but I'm not opposed to them either. It's a matter of personal choice.

Note that two egg yolks at any one time is the maximum that should be eaten. Egg white is dangerous: it is acid-forming, is too rich in protein, is indigestible, and should never be eaten raw.

Meat

I think that meat has no place in the human diet. I do not want to expound my point of view here, because most of my readers are already convinced vegetarians. If you are not a vegetarian, but would like to get more information on the vegetarian diets, the best resources available at the moment are the books *The China Study* and *The Food Revolution*.

My observations have led me to believe, and I'm not the only one, that raw meat is especially bad — even worse than cooked meat. I don't recommend it to anyone. But I don't recommend cooked meat either.

Fish

If you put a piece of fish near a piece of meat, you'll see that it decomposes much faster than the meat. The same happens inside your body. All marketed fish have already started to rot. Fresh fish doesn't smell bad.

It is an especially poor choice today, because of the heavy metal contamination of fish -- a result of water pollution. For these reasons, I don't recommend fish.

Insects

Some authors say that insects are part of the human diet, because apes sometimes eat them. Apparently, some monkeys are especially fond of ants. So maybe our natural diet would also include ants (which are apparently rich in zinc, but that's another story...). Personally, I have never tried to eat insects and don't plan to! ☺

CHAPTER 25

Compromises

Everybody is at a different step of the journey, in every aspect of life; nobody can claim perfection, your author included. We sometimes have to acknowledge where we are, while knowing exactly where we want to go, and take it one step at a time. This brings us to the topic of compromises.

What to Avoid

The foods we are meant to eat are fruits and vegetables in their natural state. When we stray from that natural diet, the mistakes we commit can either be benign or big. Here are the worst offenders, in my opinion, (besides the obvious junk food everybody knows to be unhealthy):

Bread and Wheat — Of all the grains, wheat is the worst offender, especially in the form of bread. Going against the tradition of bread has never been popular, but progressive health experts have always understood that grains are not optimal to human beings. For more information on the subject, read *Grain Damage*, by Dr. Doug Graham.

Milk and Cheese — Cheese is very concentrated, and when fermented (such as in any ripened or old cheese), it represents one of the worst foods humans can eat. Fresh (non-fermented) and made from raw milk, cheese is a little easier to digest, but still not optimal. As a cheese replacement, tofu is too concentrated and is difficult to digest.

Fish and Seafood —All fish is contaminated to some extent with heavy metals, such as mercury, whose effects on the human body are extremely detrimental, and difficult to deal with. Just one serving can contain enough mercury or other heavy metal to contaminate a person. As for seafood, we should know that animals such as lobsters, oysters, etc., are literally the filters of the ocean. A large quantity of water goes through them, which makes seafood some of the most contaminated "food" on this planet.

Spicy Food & Condiments — Spices include: black pepper, salt, white pepper, cayenne pepper, ginger, chili peppers, raw garlic, and all the foods that contain them: kimchee, hot sauces, Tabasco, etc. The consumption of spices is extremely detrimental to health (see Chapter 15). Spices irritate the entire digestive tract, create mucus (that the body produces to protect itself), and complicate digestion.

Coffee, Tea, Black Chocolate and Cacao —These contain certain substances (caffeine and theobromine) that disturb the nervous system. If a person is eating a more natural diet, these poisons have an even more disturbing effect on the system. For a raw-foodist, one cup of coffee has the effect of maybe four cups for someone eating a standard American diet. There is no room for compromise with caffeinated drinks and cacao products, which include: coffee, hot chocolate, black chocolate, raw cacao beans, black tea, green tea, maté tea, etc.

Better Choices

Steamed vegetables are certainly better than raw-food recipes and nuts in excess. *A hot soup* can be made with steamed vegetables that have been blended using a Vita-Mix or other blender. Many people find that including steamed vegetables regularly in their diet will not give you the same results as eating an all-raw diet. Personally, I still enjoy them on occasion.

Cooked roots such as potatoes, sweet potatoes, etc., are denser than steamed vegetables. They are superior to grains, but as starchy foods, they won't give you as much energy as raw foods.

Fruit goes down easily; salads can taste bland to some people, especially without oil, salt, garlic and onion. My recommendation is to make a raw dressing with tomatoes or other whole foods, blended with avocado or a little nut butter. If that is not enough, a little *apple cider vinegar* gives a lot of taste, while not being as optimal as lemon juice. Once in a while I add *dulse*, a seaweed, carefully rinsed to take out most of the salt it contains. I enjoy its chewy texture and its flavor of the ocean. Another good seasoning is *dried tomato*, soaked in advance and chopped. Make sure you find dried tomatoes without salt or sulfites. They are hard to find. (One resource is www.livingtreecommunity.com.) *Dried vegetable powder*, as explained in Chapter 15, is excellent in salads. I particularly enjoy the flavor of dried red cabbage powder. *Acid or sub-acid fruits*, such as tangerines or mangoes, can give a lot of taste to a lettuce salad.

Drinking some *hot herbal tea* is no sin if it helps you go through the cold winter. It sure can be nice sometimes. Just make sure you avoid the numerous brands that contain caffeine.

For great recipe ideas, please check out my books *Instant Raw Sensation* and *Raw Soups, Salads & Smoothies* (www.fredericpatenaude.com).

It's a Learning Process

No one I know is consistent, and it can take a lot of time to hone this diet. If you eat something wrong, don't be hard on yourself. Just observe. You are learning. Use the opportunity to watch how you feel after eating it. If you live in constant apprehension of the effects of your still "imperfect" diet, your fear upsetting your digestion and further undermining your confidence. As Shelton has said, "Those who anticipate trouble from their meals, who eat in fear, trembling and who are anxious about the outcome, will be sure to have trouble. For these things inhibit, to some degree, the normal operation of the nutritive process."

We all know there are other factors involved in health besides diet. Although it may be one of the most important factors, it is not the only one. Peace of mind is very important. We can choose to be satisfied with what we eat by not worrying about how it could be better.

BOOK BONUS: For a list of useful tips and action steps you can take now to get your health and diet to the next level, go to www.rawsecretsbonus.com and click on "Free Book Bonuses". You'll be able to print this list and use it as a reference.

CHAPTER 26

Can You Compare Yourself to Others?

Has the thought ever crossed your mind, "How come some people eat all sorts of crap and still manage apparently to stay healthy, and live long lives?"

Maybe you wondered, "Why shouldn't I do the same?" and, "Perhaps the secret to better health is all about 'moderation,' as they say."

Everyone has a friend or a relative who, in spite of eating meat, drinking alcohol, and often smoking, is cheerful, appears to be doing well, and is even apparently healthier and more energetic than some vegan or raw-foodists! We also all have a relative who died at a very respectable age (90 or older) without putting much thought into his or her eating habits.

So, the question then arises: is it actually worth it to make efforts and eat well, be different from everybody else, face the challenges associated with it, if in the end we're not going to live any longer than our neighbors who drink alcohol and party all night?

I received a letter the other day asking the same question -- one that has been asked many times by almost every natural-health seeker.

        I am married to a man who is lean, healthy,
        muscular, very moderate and he eats
        meat, flour, sugar... anything he wants
        in moderation and drinks beer too. His
        grandmother lived to 92. His father and

mother both are in their 80's and doing
very well. My parents are robust and
healthy... they are in their 70's. Everyone
around me is doing pretty well, some people
get sick... but we all have to die. I'm so
confused... Is raw really what I'm supposed
to be striving for? Do most or all raw-
foodists experience excellent health and
never get sick? Do they live LONG lives?

My correspondent condensed in a few sentences the fears and questions that many of us have. So in this chapter, I would like to clarify some points made and demystify others.

"I know someone who eats anything he wants and is really healthy."

Ok, when you all look around, what do you see? People who eat anything they want, and yet, somehow get things done, have a career, have fun, and are not going through the same diet struggles you are.

You have been attracted to the ideal of a natural diet perhaps because of some health problems, or perhaps because you only wish to live a better life. Your friends would rather die of some horrible disease rather than change their eating habits.

The question is, do you actually want to follow them? Do you really want to go back to eating just anything, and when you get sick not knowing why? And do you really think that all of your friends who indulge more than you do are, in fact, healthy?

Being fit and able to function in the world does not equate with health. How many people do you hear about who "were perfectly healthy until they died of a heart attack?" The truth is, they were never healthy in the first place; they just appeared to be healthy, but on the inside things were not functioning as well as they thought.

"Most raw-foodists experience paradise health and never get sick."

Many people have been fooled by the idea of "paradise health". They read somewhere that the raw-food diet was going to make them live to be 120. Then they hear about some raw-foodist dying and another getting sick, and they get all confused. "I thought raw-foodists never get sick!" they moan.

In order to experience "paradise health", you would need the right constitution to start with. It would probably take generations of healthful living. But who is attracted to Natural Hygiene and the raw food diet, generally? Those who experience health problems to begin with! Do these people get better? Yes. Will they ever experience "paradise health"? Possibly not.

Let's not fool ourselves. If someone is doing their best to be healthy and still gets sick, *it doesn't mean that what they're doing is entirely wrong*. They are doing their best, but often this is not enough to guarantee "perfect health". Others factors come into play: genetics, environment, past illness history, stress, emotions, etc. Diet isn't the only factor.
Attributing every health problem to diet alone is a common mistake.

To learn more about the top factors that can cause health problems besides diet, including the most overlooked aspect of a health program that leads people to failure, go to www. perfecthealthprogram.com .You will be able to sign up for an online mini-course on this topic.

"My friends are in good health"

Look around you. You will see people who eat anything they want and appear to be making it through the day nonetheless. You could think, "They are in good health." Would you be right?

Personally, I do not know anybody past the age of 50, except my natural hygienist/raw-food/vegetarian friends, who does not take any type of drug or medicine. If you are over the age of 60 and don't take any drug or medicine, you are a rare pearl!

Everybody is sick. If you've been around people long enough, you'll know it. You'll hear about their little complaints and their various health problems. The older they get, the longer the list is.

The standard American diet catches up with everybody, including centenarians. In the raw-foods, Natural Hygiene circle, it is quite rare that someone uses medicines. Many are past the age of 70 and still in great health!

My first mentor, Albert Mosséri, wrote:

> Beware: people are all chronically sick, even if they show a cheerful disposition. They don't talk about their daily misery and pains. They neither listen to them nor ignore them. Fatigue is fought with coffee, insomnia with sleeping pills, constipation with laxatives, pessimism with wine, depression with drugs and headaches with aspirin. We think that they are doing well just by looking at them, but it's not true.
>
> And those who suffer from nothing, for how long is their strong and resistant organism going to hold up? How long is it going to take before the integrity of the organs, inherited from sturdy parents, is altered by the abuse of food? It's only a question of time. The fortunate people who have strong genetics will take more time to damage and degrade their bodies than those who have inherited a fragile constitution."

Comparing Ourselves With Others Is Pointless

Do you get the point? You cannot say "that person is really healthy; therefore if I do like them I'd be healthy too." There is much more involved than just diet and nutrition.

We all inherited a different constitution. I know, for example, that I couldn't be an athlete. That's not the gift I was born with in this world. In spite of my best efforts to eat healthy, there will always be plenty of people around me who can eat junk food and out-perform me without even trying.

But everybody has something to gain from healthful living. It doesn't necessarily mean that we will all reach the same level of health, but it's worth the try, because what's the alternative? If you're reading this book you know what it is, and you know also you don't want to take that road again...

Let's Compare Ourselves to Ourselves

If you cannot compare yourself to your friends or even your relatives, you can compare yourself to yourself. Check out how you do from one period of time to another, looking at the important factors that may have influenced your health.

What are some of these changes? Eating different foods, being in a relationship or being lonely, drinking alcohol or not drinking, staying up late or getting enough rest, exercising or being sedentary, getting enough sunshine or not, etc. All these factors influence health.

You can compare yourself to yourself and come to the right conclusions. Comparing yourself to others will always lead to the wrong conclusions.

Health is a rich subject. Understanding it is a deep process, beyond the scope of casual comparisons.

CHAPTER 27

Organic Food

Is Organic Food Essential?

Organic food is not only nutritionally superior to conventional food, it is also tastier and free of the most offensive toxic chemicals that are used in conventional farming. For these reasons, and also because I support farmers that care for this earth, I recommend getting organic foods as much as possible. However, it may not be possible for you to buy everything organic, either because of your budget or your location. This will not be a major problem. The most important thing will be to find the best produce you can —whether it is organic or not.

Some people think that they are going to be healthier just by eating organic foods. They will eat exactly as before, except that they will spend more money buying everything from the health food store. But eating organic food is not a major change. It is still better to eat conventional fruits and vegetables than to eat organic bread, beans, pasta, meat and dairy.

Apparently, monkeys at the Copenhagen Zoo can tell the difference between organic bananas and commercial bananas, and are rejecting the latter when given the choice between the two. In 2004, the Copenhagen Zoo started feeding its animals at least ten percent organic products.

You, too, will be able to tell the difference between organic products and conventionally-grown ones. Some of the differences are quite obvious. Organic foods have more taste, but also more nutrients, and fewer chemical residues.

I have found that many organic items, such as apples, pears, yams, and lettuce, are either the same price or only slightly more expensive than commercially grown; they also taste much better. I always recommend organic for your staple foods. Locate a farm in your area and buy directly from them. Or join a CSA (Community Supported Agriculture) farm. This is a service that lets you buy a part of an organic farmer's harvest in advance. As items become available, you get them weekly at specified pick-up points or directly at the farm. You get the best produce imaginable at the best prices, and you help an organic farmer in the process. There are tons of projects like this going on all over North America and Europe.

To minimize pesticides, molds and fungi, wash or peel everything, organic or not. Wash thoroughly what you cannot peel. I recommend a non-toxic fruit and veggie wash that is specifically designed for this purpose. You can find this in health food stores.

BOOK BONUS: For a useful list of the 12 most-sprayed fruits and vegetables that everybody should avoid, as well as the safe commercial fruits and vegetables, go to www.rawsecretsbonus. com and click on "Free Book Bonuses". You'll be able to print this list and use it as a reference.

Quality versus Organic Label?

To me, the quality of the food is more important than just its organic label. For example, organic apples are often kept in huge cold chambers for months or even years at a time, and their quality is highly questionable. In that case I would much rather buy locally grown apples that might not be certified organic but would meet my standards of quality. The same goes for a few other fruits. For example, I buy commercially grown mangoes, which are far superior to the organic ones. The problem is that organic mangoes, at least the ones I'm able to find, are picked much too green. Their taste is unacceptable to me.

I recommend going for quality first -- not just referring to the organic label. Ripeness, freshness, etc., are often more important than the "organic" label.

Seasonal Foods

It is now possible to eat foods from all corners of the world, at any time of the year. I saw cherries on sale recently in January. To my great surprise, I met someone who had no idea when it is cherry season in our hemisphere. For people like that, food mysteriously appears in the supermarket, and they have no idea where it comes from, or how or when it is grown.

From the point of view of health, I see no problem in eating imported foods. In many parts of the world, it wouldn't be possible to eat and remain healthy without them. But there is a limit. At least stick to foods grown in your hemisphere. Avoid apples and kiwis from New Zealand during the summer, or cherries, grapes and nectarines from Chili in the winter, for example. In addition to being expensive and copiously sprayed with toxic chemicals, they usually have little flavor, and are a gratuitous distraction from other perfectly adequate regional foods.

CHAPTER 28

Eating Raw in Cold Climates

The Ideal

Having come to the conclusion that fruits and vegetables are your ideal food, you may eventually wonder if you're not also meant to live in the warm climates where fruits and vegetables abound all year round. Unfortunately for most of us, our ancestors chose less friendly climates to settle in. Most of my readers live in cold climates where a good selection of locally grown fruits and vegetables is unavailable most of the year. One hundred years ago, it would have been next to impossible for a family in Canada to eat a mostly raw fruit and vegetable diet all year round. But now we get foods imported from all corners of the world. Why shun these modern developments? A healthy diet is now possible for all of us, in spite of the steady deterioration of the quality of our food.

If you can move to a warmer climate and build your own little paradise in the sun, I sincerely encourage you to do so, and wish you the best of luck. But not all of us will be able to do this. Most of my readers probably don't plan to move to Hawaii, Mexico, Costa Rica, or Florida in the next few years, and I write with this in mind.

The winter diet of northern raw-foodists doesn't need to be extremely different than that of those living in the south. The cold weather increases your caloric (energy) needs a little bit, so all you need is a little more food to compensate. A lot of people think you need to eat more fat in the winter, but that is not the case. The extra calories you need might just come from carbohydrates, such as bananas.

Eating Locally Grown Foods

Certain philosophies, such as macrobiotics, maintain that exotic or imported foods are unhealthy. With this in mind, oranges, bananas, avocados, papayas, and mangoes wouldn't be good for Canadians; apples, blueberries and pears wouldn't be good for Indians.

If you think about this a bit, you'll realize that there is no major difference between the constitution of a Canadian and an Indian. The two belong to the human race. By the same token, you could fly to India tomorrow and eat mangoes there. Will your constitution change? Will those foods suddenly become good for you? And what if you decide to move to India? Your stomach, intestines and other organs are still the same.

I understand that the critics often address the quality of food and environmental issues related to imported foods. Of course, an imported mango isn't as good as one picked straight from the tree. However, it is still better to eat an imported mango than to eat grains that have been stored for months, or even apples that are kept for up to a year in giant freezers, before being sold. But now, due to the efficiency of our distribution system, we are getting very good quality foods. For example, some of the mangoes I can get in Montreal, Canada beat those that I've been able to buy in the countries where they are grown.

As for the environmental issues, I agree. It isn't environmentally friendly to eat imported foods. However, if I could only eat locally grown foods, I'd be forced to eat shriveled up apples and carrots for months. I simply could not eat that way. So eating imported foods is another compromise. But producing and exporting fruits and vegetables generally require fewer resources than producing animal foods or even grains. And you can still make the choice to avoid foods that have been imported from far, far away -- such as durians and coconuts from Thailand.

Food Quality

During the long winter of the north, local produce is scarce. Lettuce is often weeks old, since it has to be imported from southern farms. Thus it may be useful to buy or grow fresh sunflower greens. This sprout can actually be considered a green vegetable. You can easily grow sunflower greens in your home. Cut immediately before consumption, they are certainly the freshest and tastiest of winter vegetables.

Handling the Cold

Many people complain about the cold. Many raw-foodists give the strange advice of eating spicy foods, such as cayenne pepper and garlic. However, these foods are toxic (see Chapter 7) and simply create the illusion of heat, whereas in reality, they produce the opposite effect. When you eat cayenne pepper and feel "nice and warm", it is just your body activating its metabolism to reject the poison (capsaicin) found in cayenne pepper.

A common reason for "freezing" during the winter on a raw food diet is eating cold foods. Fruit that is still cold from the refrigerator when eaten will make you cold. It may even give you the chills. My advice is to avoid cold food at all costs during the winter. Pull from the fridge the fruits and vegetables that you will eat the next day. They need to be at room temperature when eaten. If you want to eat something straight out of the fridge, warm it up in water. For example, immerse a few apples in warm water for ten minutes. Do the same for grapes, pears, etc.

Exercise is the best way to warm up during the winter. An aerobic workout can increase metabolism up to ten percent above the resting rate. To put this in perspective, this means that if you were to work out hard for one hour while dissipating no heat at all, you could raise your body temperature to 140 degrees Fahrenheit! Your body sweats to dissipate that heat, but still, you can chase away the cold any day by a little morning workout.

Tropical Fruits vs. Temperate Fruits

There is some controversy over which kind of fruit is better, depending on its climate of origin. One theory states that tropical fruits are better than temperate fruits because our body is more genetically adapted to them. So, papayas, mangoes and bananas would be better than apples, pears and berries. However, I have never found substantial proof of this.

My thought about this is that they are equally good. Pears, apples, peaches, and cherries — these are all excellent and delicious foods, just as papayas, mangoes and litchis are.

I enjoy the variety of fruits that Earth has to offer, depending on where I am and what's available to me. Many of the most delicious fruits are not well known: cherimoya, litchi, jackfruit, durian, etc. As people eat more fruit, more varieties will become available to everyone.

CHAPTER 29

Food Supply

On a conventional diet, we do not notice the quality of our fruits and vegetables too much, since they are cooked, seasoned and mixed. On a raw food diet, getting access to a variety of good, ripe fruits and vegetables is imperative. If you are satisfied with what you eat, you won't be drawn to try other things.

It's also important to secure a good supply of fruits and vegetables. The quantities of food consumed on this diet are greater than in a standard diet. Most people don't buy sufficient quantities of fruits and vegetables because they are used to buying smaller quantities of more concentrated foods. When they run out, or have a few low-calorie foods, such as apples, they often end up eating something else.

Buy Cases of Food

It took me a while to realize this. You can't really make it on this diet unless you have a huge quantity of food at your disposal at all times. As we have seen, the volume of food eaten in this diet is much larger than the conventional diet. It doesn't make sense, practically or economically, to buy fruits and vegetables in the usual way. The key is to buy fruits and vegetables by the case. That way, you have at your disposal a large quantity of food and will save money by buying in bulk.

In Montreal, I can buy a case of organic bananas for $25 (Canadian).

That ends up being $0.62 per pound. If I bought them by the pound, I would pay around $1.30 per pound. For 40 pounds of bananas, which can go quickly on this diet, I get a substantial $27 saving when I buy a case.

I also buy other cases of organic produce and have friends and family chip in for whatever they want. To do this, I simply had to set up an account with the organic distributor. Anybody can set up a simple account with an organic food distributor and buy food by the case. Have other people join and form a little coop.

I also go to one store that I know well, which is located in the central market, to buy other cases of food. When muscat grapes are in season, I buy them by the case. When persimmons are in season, I buy them by the case too. No matter what, you always save by buying cases of fruit at a time.

Shopping Around

Unless you have an orchard and a garden, you will have to do some shopping to get good fruits and vegetables. This usually means going to several markets, supermarkets and health food stores to get the best of each. Some countries and regions have better fruit than others, but in most large cities you can find enough stores to ensure a quality supply.

Organic Distributors ⊠ The best way to get organic produce at a reasonable cost is to buy directly from distributors, the same people that sell organic produce to your health food store. Ask your health food store who provides their fruits and vegetables; say you want to start a coop. Then contact the organic distributor, and ask them what they need to set up an account with you. If they have a minimum for orders, find other friends who would like to join you in ordering organic produce in bulk.

Specialized Produce Shops — These stores are usually located in the same area as the produce market in a big city. For example, in Montreal, the bigger market is the *Jean-Talon Market*. Near that market, there are several produce shops. They order foods by the truckload and often resell it to restaurants, stores, etc.; the good thing is you can buy directly from them.

Supermarkets — You might avoid going to these, but often there's no other choice. Besides, nowadays many supermarkets sell organic food. In England and Germany I could find organic food in every supermarket. Supermarkets often have ripe fruit at discounted prices.

Farmers' Markets — The best place to buy directly from the farmers. Outdoor markets remain popular throughout the world, even after all these millennia. Get to know the farmers, and ask for deals when buying in bulk.

Exotic Fruit Shops — These shops specialize in exotic fruit and fancy items. Their prices are not the best, but you can find good stuff once in a while.

Produce Shops — These are either hole-in-the-wall family shops or supermarket-like stores where most of what they sell is fresh produce, often at very low prices. Even though most of what they sell is low-quality, commercial produce, you will often find good deals on standard items and sometimes on local and tropical fruit.

Asian Markets — Asian markets are usually found in the Chinatown of a city. They can be run by Chinese, Thai, Vietnamese, or Korean vendors. They will usually feature some exotic fruits and vegetables that you'll have to try at least once: fresh jackfruit, young coconuts, fresh durian, litchis, etc. They usually have very good deals on more common fruits like mangoes, bananas and oranges, and they seem to get better quality stuff than other markets.

People in Asian markets are usually very helpful and, unlike most supermarket employees, they actually know how to select ripe fruit. If you want a ripe durian, let them pick, because they know better!

Health Food Stores — There are many types of health food stores, so you'll have to explore to find the best ones in your area. Avoid the so-called "health shops" that look more like pharmacies than food stores, with all their jars of supplements and bottles of protein powder. Find those that sell food.

I find that most health food stores now have a good selection of organic vegetables at reasonable prices. The fruit situation is often deplorable. But still, you'll be able to get all the staples: apples, pears, oranges, grapefruits, etc. You will also find dried fruits and nuts at health food stores, but it may be better to order them in bulk.

Mail Order Companies — In North America, there are several companies that sell nuts, seeds, seeds for sprouting, and other dried goods by mail. You will find a list of some of these companies at the end of the book.

Farmers — Next to growing your own food, what could be better than buying it directly from an organic farmer? You usually get the freshest, tastiest produce at incredible prices. Ask at your local health food store where to get a list of organic farmers and CSA (Community Supported Agriculture) projects in your area.

Grow Your Own

The best way to have access to organic produce is still to grow your own. It's not necessary to have a lot of space. You can even grow tomatoes and lettuce on a balcony in the middle of the city. Sprouts can be grown anywhere.

CHAPTER 30

Fasting When Necessary

You have learned what to eat. You have learned to pay attention to various factors. You seek to eat the best foods for yourself; those that match your physiological needs and cause the least wear on your body.

However, there are times when even the very best foods cannot benefit you. In your life, each day is not the same. Sometimes you feel great, and sometimes you have worries; you are relaxed and at other times you are tense and have a lot on your mind; you may experience headaches, pain or even fever. In these conditions, even the best foods will not be digested. They may ferment and poison the body, further complicating the situation. And so, just as you must know when to eat, you must also know when *not* to eat.

Missing a Few Meals Under Emotional Stress

Shelton explains:

> Strong emotions like rage, fear, jealousy
> and worry, and all intense mental impulses,
> immediately stop the rhythmic motions of
> the stomach walls and suspend the secretion
> of the digestive juices. Fear and rage
> not only make the mouth dry, they dry the
> stomach as well. Pain impairs the secretion
> of the gastric juice. Not only do all
> strong "destructive" emotions inhibit the

delicately regulated psychic [endocrine] secretion, but even too great joy will do likewise...

Worry, fear, anxiety, apprehension, excitement, hurry, fretfulness, irritableness, temper, despondency, unfriendliness, a critical attitude, heated arguments at meals: all prevent the secretion of the digestive juices and other secretions of the body and cripple not only digestion, but the whole process of nutrition...

The practice of having the patient miss a meal, or several meals if necessary, has my enthusiastic endorsement and has been my practice for years. It is a natural and an instinctive procedure, where instinct is permitted to hold sway.

Many times I have observed angry and frightened animals refrain from eating until, after the passage of considerable time, these emotional states had passed off. I have seen cows frightened and abused by angry milk-men and have seen them cease eating and not resume for an hour or more after the milk-man had departed.

It is true that under [stressful] circumstances many civilized men and women who refrain from eating, find, indeed, that they lack all desire for food. But it is also too often true that many men and women will eat large meals under these circumstances. Psychic and vital hygiene demand that under conditions of emotional stress, eating should be refrained from. Every one of my readers will enjoy better health in the future if they follow the

example of the young grief-stricken lady
who, thinking that she had been deserted
by her lover, did not eat for three days,
saying, when the lover returned, that she
could not eat and refrained from all food
until emotional calm was restored.
     *The Science and Fine Art of Food
     and Nutrition*

Physical Discomfort, Pain and Fever

Natural Hygiene gives us excellent advice, but it may be difficult
for many to follow. It teaches us to *refrain from eating when in pain,
mental and physical discomfort, or when feverish.* Those that always
follow this rule are almost sure never to develop chronic illness,
because they always let their bodies detoxify when they need to the
most. Shelton, again:

Pain, fever and inflammation each and all
hinder the secretion of the digestive
juices, stop the "hunger contractions,"
destroy the relish for food, divert the
nervous energies away from the digestive
organs and impair digestion. If pain is
severe or fever is high, all desire for
food is lacking. If these are not so
marked, a slight desire may be present,
especially in those whose instincts are
perverted. Animals in pain instinctively
avoid food...

The absence of hunger in fever has been
shown to be associated with the absence of
hunger contractions. This should indicate
the need for fasting. Any food eaten while
there is fever will only add to the fever.
The fact that a coated tongue prevents
the normal appreciation of the flavors of
food, thus preventing the establishment of
gustatory reflexes and, through these, the

secretion of appetite juice, should show
the great importance of enjoying our food.
The feverish person needs a fast, not a
feast...

The body needs all its energies to meet
this new circumstance and it requires much
energy to digest food. Food eaten under
such conditions is not digested. It will
ferment and poison the body.
> *The Science and Fine Art of Food
> and Nutrition*

The 24-Hour Fast

Once it a while, it will be a good idea to fast twenty-four hours. This allows the digestive organs to take a rest and greatly benefits your overall health. This kind of short fast should be done whenever you do not feel entirely like yourself.

When you fast and miss a few meals, the mind clears, and all moroseness disappears. You find your balance again. The 24-hour fasts help you correct these mistakes, giving your digestive organs a short, well-needed rest. You can benefit from it from time to time.

> The 24-hour fast enables us to find our
> peace of mind and tranquility. Life's
> difficulties are not as overwhelming when
> the stomach is empty. Calm comes back and
> discouragement fades away. Enthusiasm is
> reborn and hope returns. All the miseries
> will then seem less important than they
> first seemed.
> *Albert Mosséri
> Santé Radieuse Par Le Jeûne.*

I do not recommend this fast on a weekly basis though. Fasting a day per week is the equivalent of fasting fifty-two days per year. This is a lot, probably more than you should. What I'm talking about here is fasting one day once in a while, whenever you feel the need for it.

The Occasional Two to Three Day Fast

There are times when you may need to fast for two to three days to get back your mental and physical balance. Perhaps you have made too many mistakes: not getting enough sleep, working too much, eating too much without hunger, or eating unnatural foods. Because of this, you may have headaches, pains or digestive disturbances. It may be the death of a relative (or even being in love) that makes you lose your appetite. In these conditions, you should fast for two to three days, drinking only water. This is much better than eating without hunger.

Fasting for two to three days without supervision is safe for almost everyone. When the need is felt, usually manifested by a complete lack of hunger, then you can confidently, and with relief, refrain from eating until your balance comes back. The short two to three day fast is a good way to let your body heal, recover and get a fresh start.

Stressful situations — exams, deaths in the family, stress, etc. — may require a short fast. Those who "eat their worries away" are laying the ground for worse ones, and are suffering enormously in the meantime. On the other hand, those who fast for two to three days under these circumstances quickly regain their balance and the inner power to face the situation with courage, confidence, a rested body and a clear mind.

Longer Fasts

Longer fasts are often necessary when facing more serious and complicated health challenges, or for those wanting to experience the deep rest and rejuvenation brought on by a complete fasting cure. These fasts should be supervised, not by a medical doctor, but by a competent professional hygienist who possesses both a good understanding and experience with fasting. Please refer to Appendix 5 at the end of this book.

CHAPTER 31

Where to Go From Here

Now that you've just finished *The Raw Secrets,* let's talk about where this information is going to take you from here.

Since the first edition of this book was published in 2002, I've received hundreds of letters and e-mails from people thanking me for writing it. It's really what motivated me to work on a second edition, and to make it even better.

Most people are extremely relieved to find the information in this book, after having tried different diets before; yet some people are overwhelmed by the changes they know they'll have to make in their diet. Others simply think they will not be able to eat such a "strict" diet for the rest of their lives.

At first, change is always scary. But let me tell you something: whatever is holding you back from making the right choices for your health is going to hold you back in every area of your life. In fact, it has been holding you back all your life.

If you want to enjoy different results, you will have to take different actions. And the hardest part in all of this isn't what you imagine. The hardest part is to *decide* with all your heart that you are going to *commit* to making this change. Once you do that, the rest becomes easy.

Let me suggest to you some tips and advice on what to do from here.

1) **Try a raw-food diet such as the one I describe in this book for a week or two**. You don't have to attempt to change for the rest of your life. Just try it for a week or two and observe how you feel. Then after this week, go back and read *The Raw Secrets* again for more insights.

2) **Be sure to visit www.rawsecretsbonus.com** and click on "FREE BOOK BONUSES" to receive these valuable gifts.

   - A free subscription to my online newsletter *Pure Health & Nutrition* (a $97 value)
   - A free subscription to my weekly *Raw Recipe of the Week* Newsletter (a $47 value)
   - An interview with a mother who raised children on a raw-food diet, as well as guidelines for feeding young children.
   - A series of articles on the importance of greens and green smoothies.
   - A list of action steps you can take right now to get your health and diet to the next level
   - A list of the top-12 most sprayed fruits and vegetables, as well as the safe commercial fruits and vegetables

3) **Immerse yourself in this information**. Remember that *The Raw Secrets* is only an introductory book. There is so much more that needs to be explained in order to give you the full picture. My website www.fredericpatenaude.com, as well as my online newsletter, will help and guide you.

4) **Realize that you can't do this on your own.** After having been involved in the raw movement for many years and having written extensively on the subject, I realized that this wasn't enough to help people to make some real changes. Real changes require:

a) **A high impact situation.** Just reading a book is good to open your mind, but for real changes to occur you need to find yourself in a situation that has a much bigger impact.

b) **A high frequency.** Although you read *The Raw Secrets,* and might read a few other books or information products, you need to be *frequently* in contact with this information and other information you don't even know you need.

c) **Ongoing support.** There's a saying that goes, "If you could have done it on your own you probably would have already done it." The point is that you need constant support in order to be able to succeed in a great endeavor. You can't do this alone.

Although my company mainly distributes books and informational courses, we have decided to go a step further and provide you with the necessary *constant support* you need in order to succeed not only with this diet, but also in all areas of your life.

Remember what I said in this book: "You can't change one thing without changing everything."

Starting in May 2006, you will be able to join an exclusive, Internet-based membership program called:

Raw Vegan Mentor Club

This program will help you to succeed with your health, fitness, and lifestyle goals (and other personal goals) by being provided with advanced tools and unique information.

It features:

- A growing community of health, fitness and raw-food enthusiasts.
- Access to the community forum to connect and get your questions answered.
- A monthly raw food menu planner (complete with recipes and shopping lists!)

- Exclusive audio programs and ebooks
 - A printed newsletter
 - Discounts on our products
- And more!

To claim your membership and receive over $400 worth of free bonuses, go to: www.fredericpatenaude.com/mentorclub.html

To your health and success,

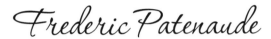

APPENDIX 1

Comments on Various Foods

Fruits & Vegetables, Nuts & Seeds

Asparagus — Asparagus contains an odoriferous poison that is eliminated through the urine. To be eaten in limited quantities.

Banana — Usually it is a staple in the raw-food eater's diet. Many authors condemn them for being too high in sugar and hybridized. These authors would like us to give up bananas and consume their jars of oils instead. No, the banana is a very good food. When fully ripe they are easy to digest, and their high-caloric density is a boon when it comes to meeting your energy needs on this diet. The fact that they are easily available makes them even more useful.

Broccoli, Cauliflower — I don't think we get much out of these vegetables when we eat them raw, because of their strong cellulose (fiber). Still, they are quite tasty sometimes. Eat small amounts and chew well.

Carob — Carob is excellent. Raw carob pods are amazing! Though carob powder is usually roasted (no matter what the package says), you can use it as a chocolate replacement in recipes. Those wanting to give up chocolate may use carob bars to help them. But read the ingredients: some companies still include cocoa powder in these bars.

Celeriac (celery root)— I love this vegetable! It is a root vegetable found in some markets and health food stores. It's kind of weird looking. Peel it and slice the inside. It's delicious and can be eaten raw, plain or blended in soups!

Celery — I've always thought that celery is excellent, especially the variety available in North America. It is salty, rich in minerals, and very delicious raw. Sometimes you feel like eating something, although it's not genuine hunger. You could chew a rib of celery instead of reaching for a piece of fruit or something heavier. Celery is very alkaline-forming.

Cilantro (Coriander) — Has a wonderful scent and aroma. However, it's not a plant you would want to eat in large quantities on its own. Some people have reported mild indigestion after eating it; it wouldn't surprise me. Use in moderation.

Citrus — Eat these fruits in moderation. There is a limit to the quantity of fruit acid the body can neutralize. That is why you have to be careful when eating acid fruits. Don't think you can eat them in large quantities. The citrus fruits and pineapples you buy at the store are more acid than those you would pick fully ripe from the tree or plant. Acid fruits are best eaten before other varieties of fruits. If you are going to eat more than one type of fruit at a meal, start with the acid fruits. Acid fruits are best eaten in the morning or early afternoon. Avoid them in the evening, especially at night. The body is tired then and will have difficulty neutralizing the acids.

Dates — The junk food of the raw-foodist. Better to avoid them, unless not enough fresh fruits are available. Dates can be an essential survival food during expeditions to the forest, mountains, desert islands, other planets, etc.

Durian — A fascinating and delicious exotic fruit that comes from South-East Asia. It can also be found at Asian markets, usually frozen. In Canada, you can also get them fresh, but they are quite expensive. At the store, you can buy whole durian or packages of frozen durian flesh. Ask them to choose one for you, if it's your first time.

Greens — All edible varieties are excellent. You should eat them regularly; about one pound per day, but it's okay if you skip a few days.

Jackfruit — This fruit is definitely one of my favorites. Too bad, this exotic fruit is not available except in Asian markets, Hawaii, the Caribbean islands, the South Pacific and Southeast Asia. Ripe, its flesh is bright yellow, with a very sweet taste and the flavor of Juicy Fruit gum.

Pineapple — Look for varieties ripened on the plant. They can be golden or green. It just depends on the variety. They are quite acidic, even when bought ripe. In the tropics, when they fully ripen on the plant, they are less acidic. Avoid eating too much (see Citrus); just a few slices are good. Notice that closer to the base of the pineapple it's actually sweeter.

Potatoes — Some authors have vehemently attacked potatoes, often with lame arguments. But eating steamed potatoes is much better than eating bread, grains, pasta, etc. They can be used during transition instead of bread. I would like to see the world eating more potatoes and less bread. Potatoes are easy to digest; they are low in protein, but their proteins are of high quality. Potatoes are alkaline-forming. They have to be cooked, but they don't have the same problems as grains. While not an ideal food, they are still far better than most cooked foods, and even many raw foods, such as complicated recipes or nuts and seeds in excess.

Spinach — Spinach contains a lot of oxalic acid that binds with calcium to form oxalates. Avoid eating it too often.

Sprouted Beans — I advise against eating raw sprouted beans. Steve Meyerowitz, the Sproutman, who wrote many books on sprouting, says, "Although sprouting makes the large beans easier to digest, increases their protein and lowers their starch, they are still primarily raw beans. Quantity and regularity of consumption is the caveat here. One should not regularly consume large quantities of raw beans or raw sprouted beans..."

Some Popular Foods and Products

Bragg's Liquid Aminos — This product is an unfermented, wheat-free soy sauce. The company says it adds no salt, but its saltiness is the main reason people eat it. The manufacturer refuses to explain how it makes it. This in itself is very suspicious. Anyway, this product comes from a factory, is highly refined, and therefore has no place in the kitchen of a truly health-conscious person. Nature does not produce any type of soy sauce.

Chocolate — Chocolate is eaten as a food, but in fact, like coffee, it is a drug. It is made from cacao beans. In both its natural and roasted state, the cacao bean has a very unpleasant taste due to the presence of several toxic alkaloids, including theobromine — a poison similar to caffeine. Camouflaged with sugar and fat, it is eaten all over the world and cherished by people of all classes. Replace chocolate with carob, or pitted dates stuffed with almonds.

Cacao (Raw) — Raw cacao beans are now sold by different raw-food companies as the latest "super-food". Cacao beans are traditionally roasted and used to make chocolate. Now raw-foodists have found a raw version of the beloved bean, and are apparently using it for its stimulating properties. I have written an article that demystifies Raw Chocolate. It can be found on my website at www.fredericpatenaude.com, under "articles".

Coffee — Coffee is a serious poison and a drug. It is blindly consumed all over the world by hundreds of millions of people who are chronically stressed by the insane demands of civilization. In addition to caffeine, coffee contains dozens of other poisons. Caffeine creates a frenetic, distressed state of mind (mistaken for alertness) as the body mobilizes to neutralize and reject it. This activity is often mistaken for energy. In fact, coffee drinking drains your energy. It's like whipping a tired horse so that it goes faster —

eventually it will collapse.

Coffee drinking is hard to give up for most people. Depending on how many cups you were used to having in a day, you may experience light or severe detoxification symptoms once you quit. They rarely last more than two to three weeks. Hold on! Have courage! To help the transition, go to www.teeccino.com. This company offers a great coffee substitute as well as tips and resources on giving up coffee.

Hot Beverages — The habit of drinking hot beverages is hard to give up, so I suggest the following hot drinks as replacements:

- Hot almond milk with a dash of cinnamon.
- Homemade vegetable broth without salt.
- Hot water with lemon juice or orange juice. Optional: ginger (boiled in water) and a touch of maple syrup.
- Coffee replacement, or Teeccino (www.teeccino.com)
- A mild herbal tea (caffeine-free).

Avoid drinking these liquids really hot. If they burn your fingers, they will also burn the inside linings of your mouth and stomach, which are much more delicate.

Miso — Miso is a very salty paste made in a factory, with cooked, then fermented, soybeans. In other words, it's not a healthy food.

Molasses — A by-product of the sugar industry, molasses contains significant quantities of iron, calcium and trace minerals. According to T.C. Fry, who created the Life Science Course, "These minerals are mostly resulting from the residues from the lime, cattle bones, soil, and other residues left after being boiled for many hours at high temperatures. Molasses is worse than refined sugar, as it carries with it all the bad qualities of refined sugar, plus the added toxins. When we ingest such a totally unwholesome and anti-life product as molasses, we are truly destroying life. Molasses should never be used as food for humans. It is a poisonous by-product in the manufacture of cane sugar and contains many contaminants and impurities."

Mushrooms — I don't consider mushrooms to be human foods. As fungi, their role in nature is to recycle certain elements. They contain few nutrients. But still, eating a few mushrooms (the edible ones, folks!) once in a while is without consequences. ☺

Nama Shoyu — I briefly used this unpasteurized soy sauce a couple years ago. But it didn't take me very long to realize it had no place in the human diet. Nama Shoyu comes from a factory and contains a lot of added salt. I don't recommend it. The same goes for any other type of soy sauce.

Peanuts — Peanuts are really a legume, but classified as a nut because of their composition. I think you can eat them rarely, though some people have stronger negative reactions to them than regular nuts.

Seaweed — Many types of seaweed come from a factory, where they have been tenderized and cooked. Some are less processed, like dulse. A danger in eating seaweeds is the levels of contaminants, such as heavy metals, they may contain. Even the organic seaweeds that are tested for these contaminants may contain them in some quantity, even though they are guaranteed to be within "safe" levels. For these reasons, and the fact that most of them contain a lot of sea salt, I advise eating seaweed sparingly.

Tahini — Tahini is hulled sesame seed butter. Raw tahini is hard to find, but you can buy it from Living Tree Community (www.livingtreecommunity.com). Other "raw" tahinis are made from roasted seeds. How much tahini or other nut butter can you consume? One to four tablespoons appears to be a good amount.

Tofu — Tofu is cooked soymilk coagulated into a bland, chewy bloc. It is rich in protein, but it contains few vital elements. It is not very tasty and is processed in a factory. It is not part of a natural diet.

Yeast — Yeast, yet another substance unfit for human consumption, is nonetheless popular as a supplement and as a seasoning in vegetarian circles. It complicates digestion by encouraging fermentation. The role of yeast in nature is to reduce plant and animal substances to the mineral state. It is not meant to be eaten.

APPENDIX 2

Menu Plans

Menu #1

A typical menu based on the recommendations found in this book could look like this (this is just a general guideline. You can be really creative still by trying different recipes):

Breakfast: Fruit, smoothies, or green smoothies.

Lunch: Fruit meal, smoothie, or green smoothie.

Early evening or late afternoon (if hungry): Another fruit meal, smoothie or snack
This can also be taken before the evening meal.

Evening meal: Vegetable meal (with or without fatty foods, such as nuts and seeds)

Menu #2 (more transitional)

Morning: Fruit, smoothie, or green smoothie.

Noon: A large salad

4-6 pm: A fresh fruit snack

Evening meal: Vegetable meal, with some fatty foods (nuts, seeds, etc.)

How it Works

I suggest exercising in the morning to create true hunger. I personally like to go to the gym or exercise in the morning, on an empty stomach. When I come back home, I have my breakfast.

For your first meal, eat a fruit (whole or as a smoothie) with or without lettuce and celery. There are several types of fruit meals that can be made. You can make a fruit salad, make a smoothie, make a green smoothie (see below), make a fruit "soup", or simply eat fruit on its own.

Lunch is also a fruit meal, but should include more rich fruits such as bananas. Personally, I will often eat fruit as a mono-meal for breakfast, and make a giant smoothie for lunch. I also might have another smoothie in the afternoon.

My favorite fruits are: fresh figs, mangoes, peaches, papaya, and some other tropical fruits. :-)

Evening Meal

The *evening meal* can be taken in different courses (one or several), in the following order:

- Fruit (ideally, late afternoon, or as an appetizer before the evening meal)
- Vegetable juice (if desired)
- Avocado, nuts, or nut butter, with some raw vegetables
- A raw soup, or blended salad
- A large salad (see below)

Thus, one day you might decide to have a fruit meal or a green smoothie (see below) in the evening, and nothing else, and that is fine. Another day you could have vegetable juice followed by a large salad. Other options could be:

Day 1
Course 1: Fruit
Course 2: Vegetable juice, with some vegetable pulp (from the juicer) and avocado

Day 2
Course 1: Vegetable juice
Course 2: Raw soup with pieces of avocado
Course 3: Steamed vegetables (if cooked foods are consumed)

Day 3
Course 1: Fruit
Course 2: A blended salad
Course 3: A large salad.

Day 4
Course 1: A fruit smoothie
Course 2: A large salad

Day 5
Course 1: Avocado, taken on an empty stomach
Course 2: Vegetable juice, with some raw vegetables

Cooked Options (if consumed):

- An assortment of steamed vegetables with some lettuce, or
- A large salad with steamed potatoes, or
- A home-made soup without salt or oil
- A large raw salad combined with steamed vegetables, or
- Any other combinations of steamed vegetables, including root vegetables and sprouted and cooked beans.

Some Comments:

- Avoid fruit in the evening, if you're going to have cooked

foods later.
- Avoid cooked foods, if you have nuts or avocado in the evening.

The Basic Raw Meals and Dishes

Fruit Meal

The idea of a fruit meal takes a little time to get used to. It is, however, the basis of the raw-food diet. Fruit meals can be taken in various ways. First, there is a mono meal. So, for example, seven or eight large bananas with nothing else can form a satisfying meal. Or a few types of fruits can be taken together at one meal. For example: one orange, two mangoes and two apples. Fruits can also be chopped and turned into a fruit salad. The possibilities are endless. Fruits also combine well with green leafy vegetables. You can also make delicious fruit soups (I give recipes in my book *Instant Raw Sensations*).

Fruit Smoothie

Fruit smoothies are a great way to take fruit in a concentrated form. This is important, because at first you will find that you are not able to eat sufficient quantities of fruit to satisfy your hunger for long periods of time. You might find that you are not able to eat seven or eight large bananas, for example. But by blending them with water and turning them into a smoothie, you might find it quite easy to drink them down! To make a smoothie, simply blend fruit with some water. You'll find tons of ideas in my book, *Raw Soups, Salads & Smoothies*, as well as *Instant Raw Sensations*.

Green Smoothie

The green smoothie is a variation on the fruit smoothie. Here's a description from an article by Victoria Boutenko, author of *12 Steps to Raw Foods*:

What do I mean by green smoothie? Here is one of my favorite recipes: 4 ripe pears, 1 bunch of parsley and 1 big cup of water. Blended well. This smoothie looks very green, but it tastes like fruit.

Green smoothies are very nutritious. I believe that the ratio in them is optimal for human consumption: about 60% ripe organic fruit mixed with about 40% organic green vegetables.

Green smoothies are easy to digest. When blended well, all the valuable nutrients in these fruits and veggies become homogenized, or divided into such small particles that it becomes easy for the body to assimilate these nutrients, the green smoothies literally start to get absorbed in your mouth.

Green smoothies, as opposed to juices, are a complete food because they still have fiber. With a ratio of fruits to veggies at 60:40 the fruit taste dominates the flavor, yet at the same time the green vegetables balance out the sweetness of the fruit, adding a nice zest to it.

By consuming two or three cups of green smoothies daily you will consume enough greens for the day to nourish your body, and they will be well assimilated. Many people do not consume enough greens, even those who stay on a raw food diet.

Green smoothies are perfect food for children of all ages, including babies of six or more months old when introducing new food to them after mother's milk. Of course

you have to be careful and slowly increase
the amount of smoothies to avoid food
allergies.

Regular consumption of green smoothies
forms a good habit of eating greens.
Several people told me that after a couple
of weeks of drinking green smoothies, they
started to crave and enjoy eating more
greens. Eating enough of green vegetables
is a problem with many people, especially
in children.

Some of my favorite greens to add to green
smoothies: parsley, spinach, celery, kale
and romaine. My favorite fruits for green
smoothies are: pears, peaches, nectarines,
bananas, mangoes and apples. Strawberries
and raspberries taste superb in green
smoothies, when combined with ripe bananas.
Victoria Boutenko
www.rawfamily.com

To learn more about the benefits of green smoothies and the
revolution how they can help you overcome deficiencies, improve
your dental health, help you lose or gain weight, and more, please
be sure to visit: www.GreenForLifeProgram.com

Raw Soup

A raw soup is easy to make. There are various ways to make it. I like
to start by blending some tomatoes or cucumber, without water,
and adding lots of celery and other mild greens, such as spinach or
romaine lettuce. I sometimes add a little avocado or nut butter, and
season with dulse or kelp (a seaweed), or simply some lime juice.
The raw soup is an excellent way to consume more vegetables. For
recipes, consult my book, *Raw Soups, Salads & Smoothies (available
as part of the Raw Health Starter Kit, www.fredericpatenaude.com/
starterkit.html)*

Blended Salad

The blended salad is a much thicker and heartier version of the raw soup. It contains more dark leafy vegetables. It's truly one of the healthiest raw-food meals you can make.

BOOK BONUS: To receive a special article on the benefits of blended salads (along with a recipe), go to www. rawsecretsbonus.com and click on "Free Book Bonuses".

Vegetable Juice

Most hygienists shun juices, but I personally enjoy drinking vegetable juices. They require almost no digestion, and are a great way to increase your consumption of green vegetables. You need to have a proper juicer, such as the Green Star (about $400), because most juicers extract very little, and generate heat in the process. You can drink vegetable juices in the morning instead of breakfast, or as an appetizer before dinner. Celery and other green vegetables (kale, spinach, etc.) are the main ingredients. Apple or carrot juice is only used as a flavoring. I personally like to add lime juice to my vegetable juice. Sometimes, I drink a little over half the juice, then save 25 % of it, and mix it with the pulp of the juice. I eat that with slices of avocado. It's simply delicious!

The Large Salad

A proper salad is a delight for the eyes. Arrange a few chopped, sliced or grated raw vegetables. Use young salad greens, lettuce, celery and root vegetables. I enjoy adding bell pepper, tomatoes, cucumbers or thinly sliced zucchinis. Top it off with a few seasonings.

Seasonings:

- Avocado
- Lemon or lime juice

- Dried tomatoes, soaked (salt-free)
- Chopped parsley or cilantro (coriander)
- Chopped green onions (not the bulb, but the green part)
- Dressing - blend tomatoes with avocado or nut butter and some of the other seasonings listed above

Steamed Vegetables

When I say steamed, I don't mean the popular method of steaming vegetables in a basket over a large quantity of boiling water that gets thrown away. This method of steaming robs the vegetables of too many vitamins and minerals. The best way is to cook in a pot, without a basket, with a heavy lid, with as little water as possible, so that there is little or no water left at the end. Any remaining water may be drunk before the meal. Steam only until vegetables begin to soften. They should remain firm and intact.

Quantities

The quantities of food will depend on age, gender, and activity levels. Younger and more active people will require more foods than older and sedentary people. Also, men will need more food than women.

To give you an idea, we can evaluate it in terms of calories.

1500 calories/day: generally fits the needs of older folks, small women, or very sedentary people.
2000 calories/day: this is usually what is required by most women with a certain, although not very high, level of activity.
2500 calories/day: this is about what a young person requires, or a fairly active man or woman.
3000 calories/day: a young, active lad will require that.
3500 calories or more per day: a very athletic person usually needs at least that amount of calories.

To put this in perspective when it comes to eating a raw-food diet, let's see what a simplified 2000-calorie diet will look like.

1st Meal: 7-8 large bananas with celery sticks: 1000 calories
2nd Meal: 5-6 large persimmons: 600 calories
3rd Meal: A large salad (150 calories), with dressing made from blending two to three Tbs. of Tahini (about 200 calories) or half a large avocado (200 calories) with some tomatoes

It comes out to be 1950 calories, out of which a little over 10% come from (overt) fat.

The example above should give you an idea of the quantities of food required to do this diet: a lot. One of the most common mistakes that people make when attempting to eat a raw-food diet is not eating enough calories from fruit, and eating too many calories from fat. It's easy to do, because we've been trained to eat dense, concentrated foods. But raw fruits and vegetables are nutrient-dense, not calorie-dense. A higher amount of food is required to get the same amount of calories (but way more nutrients.)

Dr. Doug Graham writes:

> The SAD, vegetarian, vegan and most raw diets tend to have these same three features in common: low water, low fiber and high fat. As raw-foodists we find a meal of fruit unsatisfactory because we are hungry soon after consuming it. This is no fault of the fruit. Any meal where insufficient calories are consumed will leave the eater hungry soon thereafter. We have shrunk our stomachs to the point of deformity through the continual consumption of concentrated foodstuffs. By removing the fiber (juicing), by removing the water (cooking or dehydrating), and by increasing the fat levels above 10% of total calories consumed (cooked or raw, plant or animal, fat is fat), we mimic the SAD with many of our raw

food dishes. This is surely an unhealthy practice. Both water and fiber are essential nutrients. Therefore removing them from our food must be to our detriment. And health experts worldwide agree that we must make dramatic decreases in our fat consumption if we ever hope to achieve health.

The solution to the shrunken stomach problem is to eat more volume of fruit. This takes practice and determination. Essentially, it requires that you go on a flexibility training program for your stomach, allowing it to enlarge to the point of comfortably accommodating the food volume required for a proper meal of fruit. Most folks find that within a few months they can easily double and often triple the total amount of fruit they can consume at a meal, without consuming anywhere near as many calories as they used to consume from more calorically concentrated sources.

Tips and Guidelines

- Make a large vegetable salad in advance and store it in a sealable container in the fridge for a few days. That way, you will have always access to a healthy snack and won't be tempted to eat unhealthy foods.

- Even though the types of food eaten are always the same, you can avoid boredom by varying the varieties of fruits and vegetables each day. There are so many fruits, vegetables and nuts to discover. Have you ever heard of litchi, young coconut, cherimoya, Christmas melon, Asian pear, water chestnut, jícama root, bok choy, durian, jackfruit, macadamia nut, longans or mangosteen? Have you ever tried a fresh fig? Try out a new fruit or vegetable each week, and start shopping at exotic markets.

- Acid fruits are perfect in the morning, but are to be avoided in the evening.

- Avoid fats before 4:00 p.m. This works best for most people, but of course, you can create your own menu based on your needs.

- Avoid eating late at night. Eat nothing in the period of three hours before bedtime.

- Eating one food at a time is ideal for digestion. Experiment with mono-meals.

- Some of the worst combinations you can eat are: acid-starch, such as tomato and potato, apple and bread; sugar-starch, such as dates and bread, bananas and bread, honey and oatmeal; and protein-protein, such as avocados and nuts, cheese and nuts. The habit of eating nuts and seeds with sweet fruit (especially with dried fruit) leads to fermentation.

- Avoid eating when experiencing pain, fatigue, indigestion or fever.

- Life is not a set of rules. Once you have discovered how to eat the natural diet in a way that brings you balance, health and energy, give it less attention and live your life!

APPENDIX 3

Replacements & Transition

The following ideas for replacing foods can help you either to give up something, or to find a suitable replacement for certain foods. You will notice that some of the replacement choices are cooked. Use them in your transition from the vastly more toxic foods that they replace, and for those foods you are trying to avoid.

Replace	With
Vinegar	Lemon or lime juice
Salt or sea salt	Dehydrated celery or cabbage powder (see Chapter 15)
Spices	Onions that have been cut up and left in the open air for 24 hours; fresh parsley, green onions, cilantro, dill, garlic green, dehydrated cabbage powder, salt-free sun-dried tomatoes
Bread and grains	Sweet fruit, baked bananas or plantain, steamed potatoes, cooked chestnuts, sprouted wheat bread
Chocolate	Carob
Coffee	Teeccino coffee (www.teeccino.com)
Milk	Nut milk or soy milk
Dairy yogurt	Soy yogurt
Cheese	Avocado
Pastries, jams, candy	Eat enough sweet fruit and you shall no longer desire sweets!

APPENDIX 4

Testimonials

My comments are in italics.

Happy on a Fruitarian Diet

I have been eating 80% fruit since 1980. I am now a totally committed fruitarian, since September 1999, eating only sweet and non-sweet fruits. The transition has been gradual, easy and permanent. I am 73 and my blood pressure has dropped from 200 to 140. I cleared all my prostate problems. Paunch gone. No more aches and pains. I am never thirsty or hungry. I do not have any body odor and hardly need toilet paper.

My six-foot body has gradually dropped from 87 kilograms to 80 kilograms. I want to be in a state where I do not have to cart around any more weight than I absolutely have to. I am not deliberately losing weight or adopting any strategies to help myself, except to eat the best food I can — soft, very ripe, inexpensive fruit, which the average customer will not buy.

I puree everything to a pulp with a food processor and eat it slowly with a spoon. I am getting very good at making tasty mixtures. I am an apple cider vinegar and honey freak and put a drop of these in all the mixtures. I am letting Mother Nature, through my immune system, make all the chemical decisions. I believe she is very good at it.

Jo Mazzarol
Australia

This person was overweight to start with. Overweight people can benefit from a total fruit diet, until they reach their ideal weight. However, after that, they have to introduce salads and vegetables. I often receive such testimonials, but never from a person who has eaten all-fruit for more than a few years. Improvements on this diet would include leaving out the honey and vinegar, eating some greens and most or all of the fruit unprocessed and uncombined.

Enjoying Fruit-Eating in England

Thank you for your lovely magazine *Just Eat An Apple*. It arrived on a beautiful winter's day, and I have been reading it, alternating with sun-gazing, in the rose garden of a local park.

Even in the middle of winter in England, the sun shines beautifully. In the shade the ponds are iced-over, but the fruit-eating sun-lover can always find a sheltered sun-trap.

I am enjoying a lot of local fruit — apples and pears — which are perfectly balanced for the autumn and winter seasons. There are still some wild apples to be found. They stand out on the bare branches of the trees, beautiful balls of color and life in the winter landscape.

One thing I often get asked, with reference to diet, is, "Don't you get bored?" Even on a mono-diet, each piece of fruit is unique and within each fruit exists a myriad of different flavors. If only people knew how to tune into a "simple" diet, they would find out how complex and enjoyable are the tastes within.

I find that keeping warm, on a fruit diet, even in English winter, is not a problem. It is a case of keeping one's vitality raised. If you breathe deeply and exercise enough, you will always be warm. Fruit also gives a wonderful flow of energy: you can walk all day and dance all night!

I found your magazine a wonderful accompaniment to a sunny rose garden and I enjoyed everything in it. Thanks again for enhancing a beautiful day with a lovely read.

Yours for peace, sun, fun and love,

Anne Osborne,
United Kingdom

Anne is one of the rare near fruitarians. She eats some salad and celery.

Radical Changes

I just wanted to take this moment to tell you how wonderful I feel after having been on the raw vegan way of life (100% raw) since December 15, 1999. I feel like I have the energy of a 25 year-old and I have just turned 51! People are starting to tell me that I even look younger and that I no longer have that "always tired look". A by-product of this wonderful way of life is that I no longer use medication to control diabetes. My morning blood-sugar level is around 95 and mid day it's 113. Since becoming a raw vegan, I have lost 83 pounds and I have never felt better.

Howard Fisher
Youngstown, OH

Those who are overweight are usually very happy when going on a raw-food diet. Their energy levels go up and they feel better every day as the weight drops. Thin or skinny people do not have the same constitution and tend to experience more fatigue during transition.

Dog Diet Also Works for Humans!

Not long ago I wrote you about the mostly raw vegan diet my friend fed her dog that lived beyond twenty years and endured no diseases. It occurred to me that your readers might want to know what I feel would probably be a better option for their dogs than regular dog food.

Breakfast: fresh, very ripe fruit pieces.
Lunch: Apple pieces mixed with date pieces, date/coconut rolls, figs or other dry or semi-dried fruit to provide concentrated nutrition. You may wish to follow this with grapes.
Dinner: small green salad followed by extremely well cooked potatoes (that have been cooled and mashed with avocado), and chopped crunchy vegetables or fruit-vegetables. For example: pieces of celery and cucumber and small amounts of grated carrots.

Be sure to select genuinely ripe produce for yourself and your pets. If you buy mission figs, buy the darkest, blue/black ones you can find, that have the darkest red markings. If you buy dates or date/coconut rolls, buy the darkest brown dates you can find. Medium brown date rolls are usually not as bad as medium brown dates. When purchasing yams or potatoes, buy the darkest ones you see. Like bananas, apples and plums, potatoes that have dots are preferable because dots are indicative of ripeness.

In my view, very well done yams and potatoes are superior to soaked/sprouted seeds, nuts, grains, legumes, because the baked starchy vegetables are still much less mucus forming.

I believe a 100% raw vegan diet consisting of fruits, low starch vegetables, fruit vegetables, and avocados or olives is probably best. But only when one lives in a fairly pristine environment and can absorb and synthesize important health constituents from the elements.

Although I have practiced fruitarianism and raw veganism for extended periods, I now prefer this "dog diet" for myself as well! (Note that I often include well-cooked, low-starch veggies such as broccoli or zucchini with my evening salads.)

In addition to limiting our intake of cooked products, in my opinion, our focus needs to be on reducing our consumption of mucus-forming foods, beverages and supplements.

Karen Schechet
San Diego, California

One does not have to live in a pristine environment to eat a raw food diet. It can be done anywhere. Nuts can be eaten in limited amounts, as indicated in this book.

100% Raw

After a couple months of testing and questioning, I finally took the step of becoming 100% raw on fruits and fruit-vegetables. It is simply wonderful! My fibromyalgia has disappeared and my fatigue after every meal is nothing but a memory. My family used to make fun of me after dinner since I would become so terribly tired. This went on for years! After every meal I had to lie down and regain some strength to get through the evening! This is over, after only a week on the diet.

Another thing I notice is that my memory and brain-capacity have slowly improved — maybe I'll be able to go back to school and graduate. That would really be something! Thank you all for the good work and keep it up!

Lena Buhr
Sweden

Formerly Obese

I used to be clinically obese and suffering from Hashimoto's Disease, a type of near-total thyroid failure. Raw veganism has nearly cured me of both these abominations. I am of average weight and approaching a healthy thinness (which has always been my ideal.) My thyroid continues to recover more and more, to the point where my present dosage of thyroid replacement is only half as strong as my primary dosage in 1994!

Any idea that raw veganism is a "bland", "protein-less", "monotonous", or "anti-culinary" diet is sheer misconception. All my family now insists that I become a chef — a compliment I never received before in my cooking endeavors!

Jai Krishna Ramchand
Cardiff, CA

Going Nature's Way

I went raw for only six months, several years ago. I was introduced to it by my dad, who had great results (got off his high blood pressure medications, had several cysts disappear, as well as overcoming his diabetes problem), although he did not maintain his diet. His health problems have come back and continue to get worse.

I had my first mammogram eight months ago — nothing was found. Within the last four months, a lump has developed that is just a little smaller than a golf ball. It scared me half to death at first. But at that moment I decided that I no longer had a choice if I wanted to reverse my health problems. I have chosen not to let the so-called healthcare professionals look at me. I already know what to do.

So I started my new lifestyle four weeks ago. I implement the "Ten Commandments of Health" that Dr. Lorraine Day teaches: proper nutrition, exercise, water, sunshine, temperance, fresh air, rest, trust in God, an attitude of gratitude and benevolence. I know that I will be able to heal myself. By the way, before my first experience with raw foods, I had severe migraines that made me sicker than I want to remember. Since my diet change of only six months, I haven't had a migraine.

Thanks for all the information on your website, www.rawvegan. com. I'll be checking back from time to time and referring others who want to attain health. I think your testimonial section is great support for other readers (like me).

Cindy Hatton

Arthritis & the Raw Diet

About two years ago I came down with a severe case of inflammatory arthritis, with pain in hands and feet and a badly spastic neck. The muscles there were as tight as a drum. In a nutshell: I went all raw and all symptoms went away; and they stay away as long as I don't stray into eating bread and pasta. Very coarse whole rye doesn't seem to affect me, but I don't eat much of that, either.

Since going raw, I have instructed dozens of patients in the same, simple course of action and have seen severe rheumatoid arthritis clear up in a matter of weeks. By far the biggest problem for a person with rheumatoid is the drugs they are taking. Don't ever go that route! You're only wasting valuable time, because to get well you'll have to give them up sooner or later.

Carl S. Bosco D.C.
Coarsegold, California

Looking Good on Raw

Ah, raw food. The "experts" will try to scare you. They'll say it can't be done. That it isn't safe. But it is, and ever so healthy, provided you eat a wide variety of foods. (And I've never taken a supplement, either.)

About 15 years ago, I read the book *Living Health*, by Harvey and Marilyn Diamond. It was their sequel to the best-selling diet and nutrition book of all time, *Fit for Life*. That got me started. The rest is history.

And, despite the dire prognostications of virtually everyone I knew (who are now mostly physical wrecks themselves), I'm walking taller than ever and still looking good. Oh, and did I mention feeling ever so good? And loving life!

Good Luck!
Anonymous

Infection and Arthritis Gone

I have been a raw-foodist for four months and have been cleansed from a two-year infection that the doctors couldn't clear up! Arthritis is slowly clearing up and I have more energy than I have ever had! I was just diagnosed with breast cancer in January and sure am hoping to get some statistics on eating apples to cure cancer. I've heard of cases here and there, but are there any clear statistics? It's already done so much in other avenues of my health. If anyone has other suggestions I'd appreciate hearing from you.

Jay Tudor
Sarasota, Florida, USA

As the historian Carlyle said, there are three types of lies: White lies, Big lies and Statistics. But for a book on the effect on cancer of eating a mono diet of sub-acid fruit, see Johanna Brandt's The Grape Cure.

From Junk to Jammin'!

Most of my life I was getting by on a junk food diet: burgers, McDonald's, cheese, sodas, pizza, bottled orange juice and bread with an occasional banana or an apple. I always felt there was something very wrong and unnatural about the way I was eating, but the only veggies I had been exposed to were cooked, and I found them to be utterly disgusting. For this reason I never ate vegetables.

I used to play in the woods as a boy and pretend I was an adventurer surviving off the land. This is my earliest memory about thinking of raw plant food. It certainly didn't seem appealing to eat meat, especially if I had to catch it and prepare it myself, even though I ate meat almost every day. I'd find this disturbing that the food I was eating wasn't available in nature, and I didn't grow up where fruit trees were abundant. I fell for the protein myth just like practically everyone. I had problems through all of puberty (and before and after) with depression and lack of sleep. I had the cooked food weight lifter body for a while (some people think this is a good thing but now I see it as just being puffy.) Eventually things were catching up to me.

Luckily I'd landed a job across the street from a Jamba Juice. I started drinking smoothies every day along with my taco bell, mac 'n' cheese lifestyle. I then graduated to wheat grass, which led me to reading Ann Wigmore (*The Wheatgrass Book*) and discovering enzymes. If all my food was cooked, I wasn't getting any! I'd ordered *The Hippocrates Diet* by Wigmore and a guy in the health food store recommended reading the book *Nature's First Law*. I read it and became 100% raw virtually overnight. I had maybe 3 cooked incidents during the first month and I haven't had one since, over 16 months later now and am never going back.

I stopped smoking marijuana (it's cooked) shortly thereafter simply because I got to the point where it was bringing me down rather than up. My neck, back and hand pain has been greatly reduced, almost to the point of nil. My sleep patterns are healthy for the first time in my life. My depression is history. I've got great muscle definition now. More than ever, I enjoy eating, and I have no cooked cravings. Mostly I eat mono meals of fruit followed by leafy greens (whole or juiced). It's been months since I've had nuts, seeds or sprouts (just don't get the urge) but I eat fatty fruits (durian and avocado) and young coconuts regularly.

My skin and hair are healthier and softer all the time. Tanning is a breeze. My energy levels are growing all the time. I've gotten to the point where I'm pretty much high all the time as long as I've had enough sleep (and even when I don't, quite often.) A cloud has been lifted from my body/mind and things are only getting better the more I detox the old. I no longer have "morning breath" even if I eat a lot of fruit and go to bed without brushing. Life is awesome. I recently met the girl of my dreams (yes, she's 100% raw) and am now heavily in love! I will definitely help every person I can (e-mail me if you'd like.)

Brian (viihertz@rawfoods.com)
Dallas, Texas, USA

Freedom from Asthma and Allergies

I'm an Australian living in Holland now (for the past 18 months). I have been a "chronic asthmatic" all my life, and I have also suffered from hay fever and allergies.

It was one month after my arrival here that I experienced a particularly nasty case of hives (itchy red lumps all over my body, together with severe stomach pain), which the doctors here were at a loss to explain. They told me I was just acclimatizing to Europe; their advice was that I should get "more fresh air," and take paracetamol next time I get the rash!

After several bouts of these "hives", feeling physically worn out (not to mention the unbearable pain) I saw a different doctor, who recommended that I see an allergy specialist. Well, to keep the story short, I found out that I am totally allergic to milk and all milk products (and have been all my life, the last 32 years!) The doctor also advised me to avoid all processed foods and foods with additives.

Meanwhile, I had also been doing research on my own, and found some terrific books at the American Book Centre in Amsterdam. I read about the Breath Retraining Program for asthmatics, developed by the Russian, Dr. Buteyko. He advises all asthmatics to avoid milk and all milk products, and also not to eat meat.

Well, Dr. Buteyko was completely right! A diet that includes animal foods such as meat, milk and eggs was making me sick. Suspicious of processed foods also, I gave up all the "convenience" foods I would normally be tempted to buy, such as canned food, instant soup, any and all kinds of processed food. This has meant avoiding 95% of the "food" at my local supermarket.

To my sheer amazement, within weeks of giving up all animal and "processed" food, my asthma just stopped! I would not wake up in the middle of the night, reaching for my "puffer" (ventolin inhaler) and becleforte (both immune suppressing steroids that accumulate in your body and eventually damage/ruin your adrenal glands.) It stopped attacking when I laughed, or when I walked up the stairs, or ran for the bus, like it always used to. I was so amazed and overwhelmed, because for years the doctors told me "there's no cure for asthma," and I broke down in tears with happiness.

Determined to stay a vegetarian, and being concerned about getting all the right nutrition, I continued my search. It was while surfing the Internet, that I found your website (and a whole lot of other links.)

Now I am totally free of asthma and allergies, such as hives or hay fever, and I've never felt better. I even play tennis, and absolutely love the fact that I can enjoy sport without medication.

An intelligent raw food diet is amazing. I am not 100% raw yet, but when I go back to Australia at the end of this year, I will invest in all the groovy equipment. For the moment, I am enjoying a diet high in sprouts (I grow my own), wonderful salads (with lots of yummy dressings made from my own homegrown herbs), raw fruit and veggies (especially avocado) nuts and seeds.

I am so impressed by the raw food approach that I want to tell as many people as I can. The problem is, because of all the hype and advertising we are bombarded with in this modern world, the very thought of something so simple working so wonderfully sounds hard to believe. Now I am inspired to study nutrition in more depth, and get a professional education in health, so I can contribute to the movement that I hope will become the mainstream, in years to come. I am very glad I was open-minded enough to try the "raw" experience. It has changed me, literally.

Many, many thanks to all the raw-foodists, and people who create these helpful raw food information sites. You are such helpful, inspiring, courageous folk.

Angela Jackson
Amsterdam, Netherlands

Many Ways

It is interesting how people have so many different ideas on the same subject. I have also found that mixing greens with sweet fruit is a great idea. I just love green leaves and eat huge amounts. However I don't eat nuts or seeds and very rarely have any fatty fruits. The only fatty fruit I have is avocado. I find this diet ideal. It definitely keeps you very lean.

Pam
Perth, Australia

Just Saying No in Orange County

I have been eating raw fruits and vegetables for two weeks. I started doing it for health reasons. I am healing from a variety of conditions known in the medical community as Crohn's disease, nasal allergies, depression/anxiety, eczema, and acne. Prescription drugs I have been on for many years include Zyrtec for hay fever, Luvox for depression/anxiety, and Retin-A for acne. So far on this diet, I am feeling great and have lots of energy, clearer skin, and calmer composure. My acne has mostly cleared, and there has been a 75% reduction of oil on my face. My nasal allergies have cleared, and I have completely gone off my Zyrtec. I'm finally able to wean off Luvox after 8 years. So far the diet is doing wonders. I live in Orange County, CA. I would be grateful for any people in my area for support.

Anne D
Irvine, CA

You're surrounded! Check out my online magazine Pure Health & Nutrition *for the tip of the raw iceberg there.* www.fredericpatenaude.com

Weight Loss, Strength Gain

I am a 99% raw vegan and am loving every moment of it. At 5'6", I used to weigh 150 lbs. Now I weigh 120 lbs with about 8% body fat. I love my new body and all the energy I get from raw foods. I am still doing lots of detox, but I am getting stronger every day. Love your website (www.fredericpatenaude.com).

Werner Kujnisch
Dekalb, IL

Cancer

I just started eating this way two months ago after being diagnosed with cancer. Now I am feeling better than ever. Thank you for the information you have made available to us.

Claudia
Poulsbo, WA

Leaning Into Raw

Your site is great! I became a vegan. Now I am leaning more toward raw foods. From everything I have read, it is the best choice for my health. I am having a hard time giving up processed snacks though. My family is still eating a SAD (Standard American Diet), but they support me.

Thanks for this great website (www.fredericpatenaude.com)!

Karen
Wheaton, IL
70% Raw

The information from this website is great (www.fredericpatenaude.com). I have believed for a number of years how important it is to eat a raw vegan diet. I eat about 70% raw foods and I rarely get sick. God has opened my eyes to this truth and I thank Him for it. Hope everyone comes to see this marvelous truth.

Gregory Prisco
Mahopac, NY

APPENDIX 5

Useful Resources

FredericPatenaude.Com
6595 St-Hubert, CP 59053
Montreal (Quebec)
H2S 3P5, Canada
www.fredericpatenaude.com
frederic@fredericpatenaude.com
The author's company. Resources on healthful eating. Publishes *Pure Health & Nutrition E-Zine* (online newsletter).

Dr. Doug Graham
877-4RAWFIT
www.foodnsport.com
Resources on the optimal raw food diet and fitness. I highly recommend that you attend their live events, especially *Health & Fitness Week*.

Living Tree Community
P.O. Box 10082
Berkeley, CA 94709
800-260-5534 or 510-526-7106
www.livingtreecommunity.com
info@livingtreecommunity.com
For truly raw nut butters, salt-free air-dried tomatoes and more. Family-run.

Fresh Network
P.O. Box 71
Ely, CAMBS, CB7 4GU
United Kingdom
44.8708.00.7070

www.fresh-network.com
The Fresh Network is the main organization promoting the raw food
diet in England.

Albert Mosséri

25 rue du Grand Pré
10290 Rigny-la-Nonneuse
France
Books in French on Natural Hygiene and the newsletter, *Le Bon Guide
de L'Hygiénisme.*

Orkos

0033.16460.2111, fax 0033.16460.21.01
toll free in Germany: 0.800.999.8881 fax 0.800.999.888.2
www.orkos.com
info@orkos.com
Huge variety of unprocessed certified raw, organic foods, both
common and exotic.

Raw Family

P.O. Box 172
Ashland, OR 97520
www.rawfamily.com
Victoria, Igor, Sergei and Valya Boutenko are inspiring examples for
the raw food diet. They lead seminars all over the world.

Tanglewood Wellness Center

6135 Mountaindale Road
Thurmont, MD 21788
301-898-8901
www.tanglewoodwellnesscenter.com
info@TanglewoodWellnessCenter.com
Fasting center and resources on Natural Hygiene.
Hygienic Practitioners

SELECTED BIBLIOGRAPHY

Joe Alexander, *Blatant Raw-Foodist Propaganda* (Blue Dolphin, 1990)
T. C. Fry
  • *The Myth of Medicine* (Life Science, 1975)
  • *Program for Dynamic Health* (*Natural Hygiene* Press, 1974)
Essie Honibal and T C Fry, I Live on Fruit (Health Excellence Systems, 1991)
A. T. Hovannessian, *Raw Eating* (Hallelujah Acres, 2000)
Juliano, *Raw: The Uncook Book* (Regan Books, 1999)
Franz Konz, *Der Große Gesundheits-Konz* (Bund Für Gesundheit, 2000)
Steve Meyerowitz, *Sprouts: The Miracle Food* (Sproutman Publications, 1990)
Albert Mosséri
  • *À la Recherche d'une Santé Parfaite* (Édition Aquarius, 1998)
  • *L'homme, le Singe, et le Paradis* (Courrier du Livre, 1990)
  • *L'Hygiénisme, Petit Guide du Débutant* (Les Hygiénistes, 1995)
  • *Le Jeûne, Meilleur Remède de la Nature* (Les Hygiénistes, 1994)
  • *Mangez Nature, Santé Nature, Tome 1 & 2* (Les Hygiénistes, 1992)
  • *La Nourriture Idéale et les Combinaisons Simplifiées* (Courrier du Livre, 1976)
  • *La Nutrition Hygiéniste* (Éditions Aquarius, 2001)
Paul Nison, *The Raw Life* (343 Publishing, 2000)
Frédéric Patenaude
  • *The Sunfood Cuisine* (Genesis 1:29, 2002)
  • *Just Eat An Apple Magazine*, Vol. 2 #1-3 (Raw Vegan, 2002)
Herbert Shelton
  • *Food Combining Made Easy* (Willow Publishing, 1982)
  • *Orthobionomics* (American *Natural Hygiene* Society, 1994)
  • *The Science and Fine Art of Food and Nutrition* (American *Natural Hygiene* Society, 1996)
  • *Superior Nutrition* (Willow Publishing, 1994)
David Wolfe, *The Sunfood Diet Success System* (Maul Bros, 2000)
George B Schaller, *The Year of the Gorilla* (University of Chicago Press, 1997)
Douglas N Graham, DC
  • *Grain Damage* (Self-published, 1998)
  • *Nutrition and Athletic Performance* (Self-published, 1999)
Robert Young, Ph.D., *Sick and Tired? Reclaim Your Inner Terrain* (Woodland Publishing, 2000)

Now that you've read
The Raw Secrets...

Frederic has weekly, politically-incorrect health & nutrition news for you!

<u>Are you looking for:</u>

- Exclusive interview with top authorities
and unique thinkers in the field
- Informative and thought-provoking articles
- Useful advice and tips
- The latest relevant research, not just the newest fad

You'll find all of that and more in the
Outrageous Health & Success Ezine!

All of this is absolutely free!

TO SUBSCRIBE TO MY WEEKLY E-NEWSLETTER

"OUTRAGEOUS HEALTH AND SUCCESS"

WWW.FREDERICPATENAUDE.COM